Acute and Sub-acute Toxicology

Acute and Sub-acute Toxicology

Vernon K. Brown

Edward Arnold
A division of Hodder & Stoughton
LONDON   BALTIMORE   MELBOURNE   AUCKLAND

© 1988 Vernon K. Brown

First published in Great Britain 1988

British Library Cataloguing in Publication Data

Brown, Vernon K.
  Acute and sub-acute toxicology.
  I. Medicine. Toxicology
  I. Title
  615.9

  ISBN 0-7131-2974-3

Typeset in 10/11 pt Times by Colset Private Ltd, Singapore.
Printed and bound in Great Britain for Edward Arnold, the
educational, academic and medical publishing division of Hodder
and Stoughton Limited, 41 Bedford Square, London WC1B 3DQ by
Biddles Ltd, Guildford and King's Lynn.

Preface

The ability of chemicals to cause adverse responses under some circumstances forms part of the normal events experienced in nature. Some animals utilize highly toxic venoms and some plants have developed toxic products (e.g. alkaloids, glycosides, etc.) as part of their normal physiology. An awareness of the beneficial and the adverse effects of chemicals is not the prerogative of civilized mankind but this awareness has foundations in the activities of many primitive societies. The study of the capability of any chemical product to cause adverse effects has developed into the multiplicity of sciences that are consolidated into what is termed **'toxicology'**. The enormous increase in the ability of mankind to produce synthetic chemicals, and then to manipulate some of the chemicals for different purposes, has boosted the need and the desire for a greater understanding of the inter-relationship between biological systems and chemical entities.

Many vertebrate animals, including man, are adversely affected by exposure to chemicals and a substantial number die as a direct result of the effects of chemicals. Since it is not even possible to establish with accuracy the number of humans that are killed by exposure to chemicals it is clearly impossible to make any sort of realistic estimates of the numbers of animals that are killed or even to estimate within several orders of magnitude the numbers of animals, including man, that are adversely affected by chemicals. Throughout this monograph the effects of acute and sub-acute exposures (i.e. one-off or short duration exposure) of vertebrate animals to chemicals are considered.

As a whole toxicology has developed as a pragmatic form of science and as a consequence of this there has been a ready acceptance of test methods that are convenient but lacking in rigorous scientific foundation. Toxicologists have been accused of attributing too much importance to apparent statistical respectability at the expense of important qualitative observation. In respect of acute toxicology this has been manifested as an obsessive desire to express information on the acute toxicity of any product as the LD_{50} value while ignoring other important criteria of the intoxication. This does not imply that the LD_{50} value has no usefulness or importance and in this book there is consideration of the derivation of the LD_{50} and other related quantitative data and the sensible use of this information.

This monograph is concerned with explanation of the effect of toxicants on vertebrate species, including man, but many of the principles discussed are also applicable to the interactions between chemicals and invertebrates or even plants. An aphorism applicable to acute and sub-acute toxicology is that all predictive studies should be carried out in the exact species and identical conditions to those of ultimate concern. In reality these ideals are rarely achievable and the majority of investigations that are carried out in experimental toxicology are designed to predict events that may occur in species or circumstances other than those used for the tests. A large proportion of investigations carried out in both acute and sub-acute toxicology are intended to predict what adverse effects might be expected to occur if humans should be exposed to the product but, of necessity, the studies have to be carried out using laboratory animals. Man occupies a privileged place in the hierarchy of possible species for use in investigative toxicology and opinions differ on the ethics of whether man has the right to exploit other species for experimental purposes: it is not the purpose of this book to debate this vexed philosophical point[294] but rather to draw attention to the possible alternatives so that attitudes to this emotive subject may be developed with the possibility to further research into the subject being stimulated.

The Author is unreservedly committed to the 'three R's' in relation to predictive acute toxicology. In this context the 'three R's' are defined as **replacement** of sentient animals in investigations by the use of alternative methodology whenever possible, **reduction** in the numbers of animals used when this can be done without invalidating the investigation, and **refinement** of the methods to improve the outcome of the experimentation. At this time there is not a universally acceptable alternative to the use of sentient animal models for all predictive acute and sub-acute toxicology but this does not mean that there will never be an alternative approach and toxicologists have a duty to consider the possibility of alternatives before commencing any *in vivo* toxicity test. An appreciation of the underlying theory and practice of acute and sub-acute toxicology should make it possible for investigators to optimize the data obtained by refinement of methodology and the use of minimum numbers of experimental animals.[638] It is hoped that the information in this monograph will provide sufficient information to enable investigators to encompass the 'three R's' in their experiments.

The primary objective of this monograph is to provide a balanced and detailed account of the scientific basis of predictive acute and sub-acute toxicology together with a bibliography that will enable any aspect of the subject to be followed up in the original literature. In order to achieve these objectives the principles are illustrated with selected examples but the text is not intended to be a *vade mecum* of the acute or sub-acute toxic properties of any particular products. Because these aspects of toxicology are of importance in relation to all types of products, the illustrative examples have been deliberately chosen from a broad range of different chemical types and applications.

An extensive list of references has been assembled to support and illustrate the contents of this monograph. However, no bibliography of acute and sub-acute toxicology can be complete so that readers are advised to be aware that there are many other worthwhile publications (research papers, reports, etc.) that should be consulted on many aspects of these subjects; some of these can be accessed through the lists of references in the papers cited in this monograph. Further relevant data will continue to appear as research in toxicology is a continuing matter.

This monograph has been prepared with consideration of the needs of people who are involved in the use of toxicology in relation to matters of health and safety as well as those scientists involved in aspects of research. The Author earnestly hopes that at least some of the contents of the text will prove to be thought provoking and interesting to regulatory scientists, research workers and students of toxicology and related subjects. The text should be of some assistance to anyone concerned with the design, performance and/or interpretation of predictive acute and sub-acute toxicity tests.

The Author gratefully acknowledges the invaluable help provided by various staff of Sittingbourne Research Centre; in particular Mrs Beryl Pilcher, who struggled with early handwritten manuscripts and produced splendid typed versions, and also the Library staff for being so helpful. The Directors of Sittingbourne Research Centre are thanked for allowing me use of these resources. Encouragement from many friends and professional colleagues has been most helpful and particular thanks are due to Edward Arnold Publishers for the final product.

Contents

1

Introduction

It would be naive to consider toxicology as an exact science when it is really a multiplicity of fragmented scientific principles overlaid with a large component of subjective observation. Investigative experimental toxicology is really the gathering of information in order to provide some insight into the adverse effects of products on living systems. The majority of predictive tests are carried out using various model systems and the derived data are extrapolated because it is unusual to be able to carry out predictive investigations using the target species of most interest, or even to be able to perform tests under conditions that are identical with those of most concern. Experience has demonstrated that the information obtained in this way is often adequate and this has led to the general assumption that the practical consequences of any observations or findings are really the important test of truth or, in other words, much of toxicology has developed as a pragmatic rather than a theoretical branch of science.

In this monograph only acute and sub-acute aspects are considered and then only the importance of toxicity in relation to vertebrate animals. Some of the same principles may also be applied to invertebrates and to plants. Many acute and sub-acute toxicity investigations are carried out with the intention of predicting hazard to man but it is important to be aware that some investigations are intended to provide information on the potential toxicity of products to other animals and these may be associated with safety (e.g. hazard to domestic animals or wildlife) or with the development of intentional toxic properties (e.g. rodenticides and avicides).

Occasionally there are multiple interests in the same chemicals as for example some blood anticoagulants. The use of anticoagulants as rodenticides is long established and yet the same products (e.g. Warfarin) are used in human clinical medicine for the control of blood clotting; but the acute toxicity of the same anticoagulants may be a serious problem in terms of intoxication of predators. Owls may eat rodents that have ingested anticoagulant baits or domestic and non-verminous animals may be tempted to eat bait that has been set to kill vermin. The trend towards producing more potent anticoagulants for use as rodenticides has not been devoid of adverse environmental impact. Clearly no toxicologist can dismiss the acute toxicology of chemicals, such as anti-coagulants, in terms of facile quantitative measurements.

1.1 Some Definitions

There are some poorly defined but widely used conventions associated with what is, and what is not, classified as being toxicology. Water may be used as an

1

illustrative example of the use of the conventions. Water is a component of all living animals and forms an essential part of the nutritional requirements of vertebrate species; insufficient water intake leads to impairment of essential bodily functions and death. The amount of water required by an animal is dependent on adaptation and ambient conditions. By convention this aspect of exposure to water would be classified as being physiological or nutritional and would not be referred to as being a toxicological characteristic. However, under some circumstances water can induce severe adverse effects when imbibed[1] and some investigators have even succeeded in quantifying lethal doses of water in laboratory rats[2], thus it is conventional to accept that it is the toxicology of water that is being considered in these situations. But there is yet another aspect of the same subject; many animals die from drowning in water, certainly far more than die from intoxication due to imbibing water and, although there may be some parallels with inhalation toxicity, it is usual to classify drowning as being a traumatic death rather than a toxic manifestation.

The use of conventions in science is not uncommon but conventions can leave a sense of uncertainty about the validity of the assumptions that have led to their development. The possible mechanistic parallels between drowning and inhalation toxicity were mentioned but it was stated that conventionally drowning is not a toxic phenomenon; elsewhere in this monograph the importance of the aspiration of products from the alimentary tract into the respiratory tract is discussed and conventionally aspiration of this type is accepted as being part of toxicology. At first sight the foregoing may seem to be pedantic and of little consequence to the study of toxicology, but that is not so, for any toxicologist should be aware of all of the ramifications of toxic response to any product. To illustrate this point the commonly used fuel kerosene provides a good example. Kerosene is generally reported to have a very favourable acute toxicity rating (n.b. the acute oral LD_{50} values for both rats and rabbits are generally quoted as being about 28 000 mg kg^{-1}) and yet this 'safe' liquid fuel has been the cause of a very large number of deaths, particularly among children, throughout the world[3-5]. Although there may be some toxic manifestations resulting from systematically absorbed kerosene it is the pulmonary damage resulting from aspiration that is the primary cause of death and logically this must diminish the importance of the LD_{50} values as an index of the acute toxic potential of kerosene.

Systemic effects in toxicology are distinguished from local or topical effects. Systemic toxicology is a function of the toxicant causing effects after absorption into the organism. There are conventions used in the terminology and some examples may help to clarify these conventions. Caustic acids and alkalies (e.g. sodium hydroxide) can damage tissues on contact: this corrosion is an acute effect but it is not classified as being systemic. If the same caustic agent was ingested there would be corrosion of the lips, buccal cavity, oesophagus, etc. as the chemical passed down the alimentary tract and this could be termed a systemic effect, because it is within the organism, but this definition is not precise and is unacceptable as no absorption of the alkali has been involved in the response. Cicatrization of the alimentary mucosa may remain as a long-term effect of ingestion of sub-lethal amounts of corrosive toxicants[625]. Phenol also causes corrosive tissue damage on contact and if swallowed, phenol directly damages the lining of the alimentary tract and additionally, it causes real systemic toxic effects, sometimes resulting in death, because it is readily absorbed from the alimentary tract[6].

To recapitulate, the term 'systemic toxicity' should be restricted to toxic effects that occur only after absorption but sometimes the term is misapplied to surface effects resulting from contact with a toxicant within the body (i.e. direct effects on the linings of the alimentary, respiratory or other tracts). The distinction between direct and indirect effects is important as the indirect influence of absorbed chemicals on the externa or on tract linings of an animal may be part of the symptomatology associated with the toxicant and cannot be disregarded. For example, the hair loss associated with sub-lethal acute exposure to some thallium compounds is a clear case of a systemic effect that is apparent in the externa of intoxicated animals[646].

Within the context of toxicology use of the term 'acute' is also subject to convention. The word 'acute' implies short-term or sharp and could be used to describe either the exposure or the response. Acute responses sometimes result from repeated exposure to a chemical and are most often attributable to sensitization or anaphylactic reactions[7,8]. Generally the reaction of humans to one bee sting is limited to localized pain and discomfort but some exposed people become sensitized to bee venom and any subsequent exposure of these individuals to a further bee sting may cause a profound anaphylactic response possibly resulting in death[639]. Even some simple chemical molecules can induce various forms of sensitization reaction. For example, some of the fluorohydrocarbons that were once commonly used as aerosol propellants were not by conventional criteria particularly toxic (i.e. they have favourable LD_{50} values) but these propellants were found to sensitize the hearts of some exposed people so that the physiological release of adrenalin, brought about by any subsequent stress, could prove fatal[9,10].

The more common usage of the term 'acute' in toxicology is as a descriptor of exposure rather than response. Unless otherwise indicated the term 'acute' is used in the sense of exposure rather than response throughout this monograph. It is necessary to define the meaning of acute exposure: an acute exposure may be one-off (i.e. single) or alternatively, multiple exposures within a defined short time-span[11]. The usually accepted maximum time-span for an exposure to be 'acute' is 24 hours[12] and that is the convention used throughout this monograph.

Both multiple exposures and continuous exposure over a short time-span, but in excess of 24 hours, are referred to as being either 'sub-acute' or 'sub-chronic' exposures. The choice between the use of 'sub-acute' or 'sub-chronic' is arbitrary and largely falls to being a matter of individual preference. The dividing line between when sub-acute (or sub-chronic) becomes 'long-term' is often blurred but it is now generally accepted that sub-acute or sub-chronic exposures extend over a period not exceeding 10% of the target species life-span[680].

In toxicology the terms **dose** and **exposure** are often used interchangeably. Although the two terms are not strictly synonymous the interchange is permissible. The term **dose** implies a deliberate exposure whereas **exposure** infers a situation that may be either deliberate or non-deliberate (i.e. accidental or adventitious) in form. The definition of a **dose** generally takes the status of a specified quantity whereas an **exposure** may be more difficult to quantify. For example, an animal may be given a single dose of 10 mg kg^{-1} of a chemical (n.b. the terms **dose** or **exposure** would both be legitimate) but another animal might be exposed to an atmospheric concentration of 100 ppm for 1 hour of the same chemical, this would be an **exposure** but the term **dose** is inappropriate. Since the term **exposure** embraces **dose** but the converse is not true, the choice of word for any particular set of conditions may depend on personal preference or shades of meaning.

It is a common misconception that acute toxicology is only concerned with death as an outcome of the exposure. This idea has been fostered by a long established predilection for the quantification of data and the consequential convenience of the term 'LD_{50} value'. Acute toxicology is concerned with all effects resulting from acute exposure to products; generally it is the adverse effects that are of most concern in toxicology but beneficial effects may also be important. Death is only one manifestation of acute intoxication and there are many sub-lethal effects that are of enormous toxicological importance. Responses to the effects of toxicants can be defined as being either 'signs' or 'symptoms'. Together the signs and symptoms are referred to as the 'symptomatology of intoxication'. These important terms need definition:

Intoxication – Intoxication is a useful and satisfactory word to indicate poisoning by any product. Common usage, that has been accepted by many dictionaries, associates the word intoxication specifically with the responses associated with imbibing beverages containing ethanol. Throughout this monograph intoxication is used in the former, wider, sense.

Signs – Signs are overt effects following intoxication that can be seen or heard by observers. Such events as tremors, convulsions, noisy breathing and other visual and sound effects are all classed as signs.

Symptoms – Symptoms are the covert effects that are not apparent to observers but are sensed by the intoxicated individual. Pain and blurred vision are common symptoms of intoxication as are numerous other sensations.

Symptomatology – Despite its obvious derivation the term symptomatology is used to describe the totality of signs and symptoms. Thus a description of the symptomatology of intoxication includes a description of the observed signs together with any symptoms reported by the exposed individuals.

One of the major short-comings of predictive toxicology carried out using animals is the inability of species, other than man, to communicate symptoms to the investigator. This inability to communicate symptoms by animals is a difficulty that is well known to veterinarians in clinical practice. Details of the symptomatology associated with exposure to some products may be incomplete if the only information available is based on experiments using animals; it is very important that information about symptoms is reported for products whenever human exposure experience becomes available. The gathering of information on the toxicology of any product must never be considered to be complete, the compilation of information is a continuing process.

The short-coming of *in vivo* experimentation using laboratory animals in respect of symptoms may be obvious but *in vitro* test methods are also unable to provide information on symptoms of intoxication and *in vitro* methods are also deficient in information on signs of intoxication.

1.2 Objectives of Acute and Sub-acute Toxicity Testing

The data generated by research and investigations in acute toxicology finds applications in both human and veterinary clinical medicine, environmental hygiene, ecotoxicology, the development of new products, such as therapeutic agents, pesticides, industrial processes etc., as well as the establishment of safety criteria for various purposes such as storage and transportation. Predictive toxicity testing is frequently carried out for the purpose of predicting adverse effects of products to man but not all toxicity testing has this objective and there is a need for predictive testing in order to establish the potential toxicity of some products to domesticated animals and wildlife. Quite apart from the establishment of safety factors, some toxicity testing has the opposite objective, this is found in the development of rodenticides, avicides and also the development of agents for chemical warfare and related use where the research is deliberately seeking selective toxicity to some vertebrate species.

The four main purposes for predictive acute and sub-acute toxicity testing are:

(i) to assess toxic potential
(ii) to aid the prediction of hazard
(iii) to generate data for use in risk–benefit assessments
(iv) to provide information on the mechanisms of acute toxic action

In addition, information obtained from sub-acute tests are often useful in the design of long-term and chronic toxicity tests.

Hazard and risk are two subjects that are closely related to the purpose of acute and sub-acute toxicology testing. Hazard is the potential for the occurrence of an adverse effect under specific conditions whereas risk represents the probability of the hazard being achieved[13]. In addition to toxicity there are many other hazards associated with chemical products (e.g. explosiveness, flammability, etc.) but these are only considered here in as far as they impinge on the toxic potential of any product.

In order that any predictive toxicology testing should be as meaningful as possible it is essential that adequate attention must be given to the objectives of the testing and the experimental design. Well designed experiments often provide valuable information on mechanisms of toxic action and in turn this information may be of value for the development of antidotes or it may provide information that will be helpful to those concerned with the pharmacology of the product or its formulation. Regrettably, predictive acute and sub-acute toxicity tests are too often carried out with insufficient attention to detail and this approach must be deplored.

There must be awareness of the possibility of erroneous information arising out of the chemistry of products being tested. Impurities may significantly influence the toxicology of products being tested and physical or chemical interactions between the components in formulations may be critical to the outcome of toxicological investigations. Attention to detail in respect of the chemical criteria is essential[113-149] and this must not be overlooked when toxicants are presented in admixture with food[26-40].

1.3   The Emotive Issue of Acute Toxicity Testing

Although acute toxicity testing is firmly entrenched as part of the ritual of acquisition of information on the toxicology of chemical products there are no realistic means for determining whether the benefits accruing from all of the effort put into testing are justified or not. It is sometimes mooted that all knowledge is useful and its acquisition is justifiable on those grounds alone. The majority of predictive acute toxicity testing involves the use of laboratory animals and the ethics of such experimentation is highly controversial. Although different there is also controversy associated with the use of humans for experiments in acute toxicology. As yet there are no satisfactory *in vitro* methods capable of replacing all of the *in vivo* acute toxicity tests that are now carried out. What is certain is that despite all the acute toxicology investigations that have been carried out there is still a horrifying incidence of accidental and deliberate intoxication of man, and other animals; acute intoxications occurs not only with the obviously dangerous chemicals but with such simple everyday things as common salt[14,15] and it is not only ubiquitous synthetic chemicals that present a problem but also some of the highly toxic molecules that occur in nature[16].

Whenever predictive acute toxicology data are derived in the laboratory it is essential to be aware of the need to use the information with care. Meaningful extrapolation of predictive data is not simple and the process must take cognisance of all of the factors that may affect the situation. Although there may be a justifiable need for quantification in predictive acute toxicology it is morally wrong and scientifically unjustifiable to use unnecessarily large numbers of experimental animals solely for the purpose of quantification; investigators must always review the objectives of studies and design the experimentation to minimize suffering and maximize the usefulness of the results. The use of excessive numbers of experimental animals in any aspect of toxicology is morally wrong, scientifically unjustifiable and makes economic nonsense. This monograph is intended to clarify the major principles underlying acute and sub-acute toxicology hence providing a basis for the implementation of realistic experimental design and aiding the interpretation of data obtained from these two types of predictive toxicity tests or comparable information from other relevant sources.

2

Some Theoretical and Practical Aspects

Predictive toxicology combines aspects of theoretical biology with practical compromise and justification of the outcome is esentially pragmatic. In this chapter some of the major theoretical and practical aspects of predictive acute and sub-acute toxicity testing are discussed.

As is usual in science the speciality has developed a number of terms that form part of the language of the subject. Some of these terms are adaptations of terms used in related branches of science. Two such terms are **toxicodynamics** and **toxicokinetics** both of which are semantic modifications of pharmacodynamics and pharmacokinetics, terms that are familiar to pharmacologists and practitioners of human and veterinary medicine[17].

2.1 Toxicodynamics and Toxicokinetics

A toxicant can be any product acting in an adverse manner within an organism. If a toxicant is a chemical that is not normally associated with the physiological make-up of the organism it is classified as being a xenobiotic but it must be understood that even chemicals that do form part of the normal physiological chemistry of an organism (e.g. water[1,2], sodium chloride[15], etc.) may sometimes behave as toxicants. Any chemical entering an organism must have some effect on that organism, and an effect may be beneficial (nutritional or therapeutic), physiological (adaptive) or harmful (toxic).

Toxicodynamics describes the mechanism of toxic action of a substance and is really the totality of the biochemical and the pharmacological effects of the toxicant in the exposed organism whereas **toxicokinetics** describes the absorption, distribution, biotransformation and excretion of the toxicant by the exposed organism. As a generality toxicology is most concerned with the adverse or harmful effects of products but toxicologists must never neglect the importance of beneficial (nutritional and therapeutic) and physiological (adaptive) effects. The distinction between adverse and beneficial effects is often only a matter of degree rather than kind and what may be a desirable pharmacological property under one set of circumstances may be a situation of toxicity under other conditions. Both acute and sub-acute toxicity are sometimes associated with excessive exposure to a product and the magnitude of the exposure may cause symptomatology of intoxication that appears to be quite distinct from the pharmacological response to lower exposure rates[603]; this is often the situation with therapeutic agents. The relationship between the acceptable or desirable response to exposure and the toxic response may be critical and the information derived by predictive acute toxicity testing may form part of the essential risk/benefit analysis that is frequently applied to products (see Chapter 5).

In toxicology the word **target** is used in two distinct ways. Firstly there is the **target organism** and secondly the **target system** within the organism. The target organism is the defined animal or animals that will be affected or exposed to the toxicant. The level of definition of the organism may vary from situation to situation and in the context of toxicology may be heterogeneous or may be very specifically defined. Under laboratory conditions testing is often associated with a high level of specificity as for example by the use of a genetically defined strain of rodents under near ideal conditions of husbandry, whereas in investigations involving human exposure heterogeneity is immediately apparent (genetic variability, health status, etc.).

Targets within any organism can be considered as being of three types:

(a) functional biochemical processes,
(b) physiological systems,
(c) morphological form,

but, because of the complexity of the interactions within any vertebrate species, it is never possible to be certain that the response to a toxicant will be restricted to (a), (b) or (c) and generally toxic effects are a combination of responses exhibited by more than one type of target. In the design of therapeutic agents the objective is to be very specific about the target, or targets, but in situations where acute toxicity occurs it is common for the targets to be swamped by the toxicant; thus in acute or sub-acute intoxication   the pharmacokinetic associated with therapeutic dosage may be over-burdened[18,19,603,665]. Although the same principles apply as for therapeutics, many of the products that are of

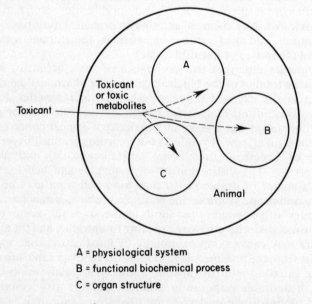

A = physiological system

B = functional biochemical process

C = organ structure

Fig. 2.1 A simple model in which the toxicant–target interaction is limited.

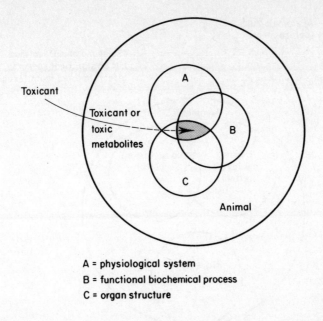

A = physiological system
B = functional biochemical process
C = organ structure

Fig. 2.2 A simple model in which the toxicant–target interaction is interrelated.

interest to toxicologists are not intended to interact with vertebrate targets but there is always the possibility of exposure occurring. Exposure may be deliberate, accidental or adventitious and sometimes there is an overlap between the various types of exposure that may have occurred in any situation involving intoxication.

The theoretically most simple situation[663,665], hence one that is unlikely to occur, is illustrated in Figure 2.1. In Figure 2.1 the target organism is shown as being exposed to the toxicant and the toxicokinetics of the product are such that it only affects one of the receptor sites within the organism. Figure 2.2. is likely to represent a more realistic intoxication but the actual amount of the receptor target complex (shown as the shaded area in Figure 2.2) depends on the particular toxicant and on the exposed species. As an aid to visualization, Figure 2.3 demonstrates, in the same diagrammatic format, the situation that occurs if the target species, in this case, man, is exposed to a therapeutically acceptable dose of the analgesic drug paracetamol (acetaminophen). If the dose of paracetamol is increased to a level that is acutely toxic then the pattern of events is better illustrated by Figure 2.4; the resultant effect (shown as the shaded portion in Figure 2.4) is likely to be death[20] [Note: the toxicology of paracetamol has been deliberately simplified here].

In order to achieve a reasonable understanding of the mechanism of toxic action of any chemical it is very desirable to establish the critical amounts of toxicants (i.e. the parent molecule and its metabolites) at receptor sites[666]. For many toxicants there will be an incipient body-burden stored in tissues (e.g. lipophilic chemicals stored in body fat; heavy metals in bone, etc.) but capable of being released and circulated to critical targets[667]. Analyses of blood for

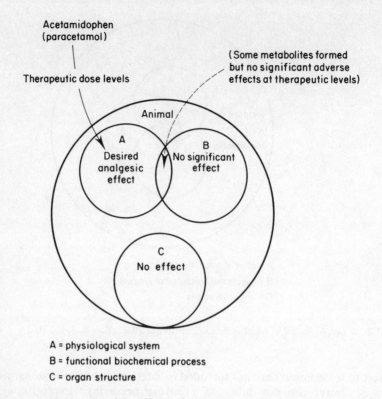

A = physiological system
B = functional biochemical process
C = organ structure

Fig. 2.3   A simplified model of the effects of therapeutically acceptable doses of
acetamidophen in man.

concentrations of toxicants can be a useful tool in toxicology[681] but it must be
realized that the relationship between circulating levels, depot levels and critical
target levels needs careful and very detailed assessment[665,682].

An additional complication to the use of the term 'target' needs some
explanation. Many drugs are used for the treatment of infections and some
pesticides are used for the treatment of infestations by endo- and ecto-parasites
that are associated with vertebrate hosts. In these situations it would be correct
to classify the infecting, or infesting agents as being the target species. Thus, for
example, if an ectoparasiticide is being used to kill ticks on cattle then a parasito-
logist would consider the ticks to be the target species whereas toxicologists are
more concerned with the cattle as the target for toxic response. In reality this
seldom causes confusion and the relevant target is generally obvious.

It has been stated in Chapter 1, that within the context of toxicology the two
terms, 'dose' and 'exposure' are often used interchangeably but that there may
be shades of difference in their meanings. These small semantic differences may
make the choice of one or other word more appropriate. Essentially a 'dose' is
the amount of a product administered or received at any one time or in any one-
off situation, whereas an exposure is subjection to the influence of a product

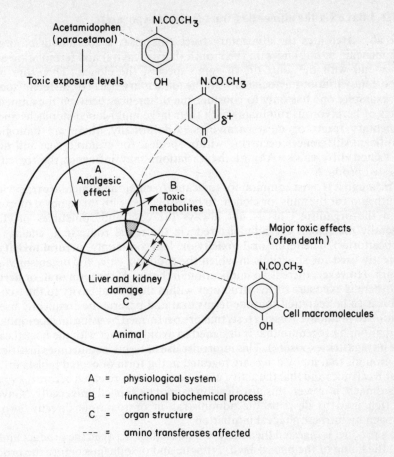

A = physiological system

B = functional biochemical process

C = organ structure

--- = amino transferases affected

Fig. 2.4 A simplified model of acutely toxic doses of acetamidophen in man.

and implies a more continuous process than is signified by dose. To illustrate this idea of shades of meaning, a single amount of a toxicant administered by any route may correctly be called a dose whereas the continuous inhalation of a vapour over a period of time is more obviously an exposure. However, it is not wholly incorrect to refer to the former as being an exposure and the latter as a dose.

In sub-acute toxicology the same use of the words applies. It is more usual to refer to a dose of, say, 10 mg kg^{-1} day^{-1} but to refer to an exposure of, say, 100 parts per million (ppm) in the diet, atmosphere, etc.

2.2 Routes of Exposure

In toxicology it is usually accepted that there are four main routes by which a toxicant can enter into the target organism. Here each of these routes is considered separately but it is important to appreciate that more than one of the routes may be implicated in some exposures.

2.2.1 Intake via the alimentary tract (enteral exposure)

For all vertebrates the alimentary tract comprises a continuum of organs, commencing at one end with the mouth (buccal cavity) and terminating at the other end with the anus or, in some species, the cloaca. There are many important variations associated with the alimentary tracts of different species, for example, one has only to consider the differences between the alimentary tracts of herbivorous ruminants with their large multi-lobed stomachs and the alimentary tracts of most carnivores. Additionally, there are biologically significant differences occurring within species, for example, age and health associated differences. Any of the variations may influence the toxicity of ingested products.

Although it is most common for toxicants to enter the alimentary tract via the mouth and for the anus, or cloaca, to be associated with the removal of excreta from the organism, this is not always the case and sometimes products, generally medicinal, are administered via the rectal route (e.g. enemas and suppositories). The terms **oral toxicity** or, less commonly, **peroral toxicity** are correctly used for situations in which the products enter the organism via the mouth. However, there is an implication in the use of the term **oral**, or **peroral**, that there is exposure of the structures within the buccal cavity to the toxicant and it is to be regretted that the terms oral and peroral are frequently used in relation to predictive toxicity tests that are performed by using intraoesophageal intubation, a procedure that is designed to avoid contact with the buccal cavity (i.e. intragastric exposure). This imprecise use of terms is sometimes justified on the grounds that many drugs are ingested in the form of coated tablets or hard gelatin capsules and that the active ingredients are not released before they reach the stomach, however, this justification cannot be applied universally. 'Gavage' is often used to describe the administration of toxicants directly into the stomach by introesophageal intubation.

If a product is ingested then there will be contact between the product and the lips, the lining of the buccal cavity, tongue and oesophagus before the product reaches the stomach. If the ingested or imbibed material is corrosive there will be contact damage to the tissues and this can be of toxicological importance; many cases of clinical intoxications are associated with corrosive substances[625]. The buccal cavity may have an important role in the toxicology of some products whereas, with the exception of response to corrosive materials, the oesophagus only has a passive role in the passage of materials along the alimentary tract. Absorption of some chemicals occurs within the buccal cavity although absorption is generally limited to unionized lipid-soluble compounds[21-23]. The ideal lipophilic characteristic for maximum buccal absorption lies within the range 4.2 to 5.5 for the logarithm of the *n*-octanol/water partition coefficient[22] and mathematical models for the investigation of buccal absorption phenomena have been developed[24].

Chemicals that have been absorbed from the buccal cavity do not wholly pass through the liver and thus hepatic toxification or detoxification will not be complete and the unchanged toxicant may reach the target system more rapidly than would occur with absorption from other parts of the alimentary system[25,632]. Some chemicals administered by intragastric gavage are poorly absorbed or rapidly metabolized within the stomach (e.g. glyceryl trinitrate, isoprenalin, etc.) but these same chemicals may be pharmacologically active if absorbed from the buccal cavity[26], a property that is utilized in their therapeutic presentation but could easily be missed in a conventional predictive acute toxicity investigation involving only administration by intubation[632].

Although there are important exceptions associated with the physiology of some classes of vertebrate animals (e.g. ruminants, birds, etc.) there are some useful generalizations that apply to the absorption of most toxicants in the majority of vertebrate species[27-29]:

(i)   Membrane permeability is directly related to the lipophilic characteristics of undissociated molecules of the chemical[618] and further it is inversely related to the molecular size[44].

(ii) Toxicants that are weak acids exist largely in unionized form in the presence of gastric acid. These unionized weak acids are much more readily absorbed from the stomach than are bases or strong acids[26-29].

(iii) Toxicants that are weak bases and exist in the unionized form in the alkaline contents of the intestinal lumen are much more readily absorbed than are acids or strong bases[26-29].

(iv) Molecules that are highly ionized are not generally absorbed from the gastro-intestinal tract unless some specific ionic transportation mechanism exists for the particular ions[26-29].

Caution is always essential when considering toxicological processes in terms of generalizations. Consideration of the ionization characteristics of toxicants in isolation can lead to some surprises in relation to gastro-intestinal absorption. For example, because the membrane carries a high charge density[30] the pH at the surface of a membrane is likely to be quite different from the pH of the fluids bathing the membrane and this, in turn, may affect the state of the toxicant at the actual site of absorption.

After the buccal cavity and oesophagus the next major organ met by an ingested toxicant is the stomach. A feature that is common to virtually all vertebrates is the fact that the contents of the stomach are acidic. It is important to be aware that the pH of stomach contents varies considerably between species and even for individuals within a species. There can be significant variation in the pH of the contents in different gastric regions within individuals[31] and these may be influenced by the state of the gastric contents hence it is important to consider the timing of toxicant ingestion in relation to food intake.

Significant absorption of some toxicants occurs within the stomach[32,33] and this, in its turn, may be affected by the rate of gastric emptying which is influenced by the nature and quantity of the contents; the toxicant itself may influence gastric emptying[34-36]. The influence of toxicants on gastric emptying varies, at least quantitatively, between individuals[37] and this alters the toxico-kinetics and influences toxic potential. For example, some of the anti-depressant drugs commonly used in clinical practice (e.g. amitriptyline, imipramine, etc.), and not uncommonly used in attempted suicides, slow gastric emptying; this retardation of gastric emptying is of importance in relation to treatment of the intoxication. There are other chemicals (e.g. metoclopramide, domperidone, etc.) that stimulate gastric emptying and small intestinal transit.

Awareness of the importance of gastric contents in toxicokinetics is important in predictive acute and sub-acute peroral toxicology[619,620]. It is common practice in predictive acute peroral toxicity tests to withhold food from the experimental animals for a period of several hours before administration of the test product[619]. The underlying logic of withholding food is the simplistic assumption that an unknown gastric content would variably influence the efficiency of absorption[38] but, although this assumption is correct, it has to be set against the fact that withholding food causes physiological changes that may affect the apparent acute toxicity of some products[39,40,620].

Within the intestinal tract many toxicants are absorbed by simple passive diffusion with lipid solubility largely dictating the speed of passage across the intestinal epithelium[41,42]. The degree of ionization of the toxicant is also an important limiting factor for absorption; weak electrolytes cross the barrier mainly in non-ionized form whereas organic anions and cations penetrate intestinal epithelium much more slowly than penetration by lipid soluble, unionized, organic molecules[43]. Gastrointestinal absorption of macromolecules is generally poor although some absorption of macromolecules can occur, but this is generally more efficient in neonatal animals than in adults[44]. In toxicology this is important as some macromolecular toxins are absorbed in sufficient quantity to cause acute effects even though the dose required to produce a response may be greatly in excess of that needed to produce the same toxic effects experienced with parenteral exposure (e.g. Botulinus toxin)[600-602].

Active transport of some molecules across the barrier occurs within the intestines. The mechanism of active transport depends on energy being provided for the transfer from regions of low electrochemical potential to regions of higher potential. This transfer, by means of active transport, is commonly observed with some sugars and some substituted pyrimidines in the normal processes of physiological biochemistry but it is also known to occur with some xenobiotic chemicals. Some toxicants form temporary complexes with biochemical carriers at the surface of the intestines and this complex formation increases either the amount or the rate of absorption without the influence of electrochemical potential. Absorption associated with complex formation is described as 'facilitated diffusion'. Saturation of carrier systems can occur and this is one of the rate-limiting steps in the alimentary absorption processes.

Lipid soluble chemicals may dissolve in fats and then be absorbed via the lymphatics[45]. In investigative acute toxicology it is common practice to dissolve lipid soluble products in various oils for peroral administration and it must be appreciated that, although the absorption characterization of different oils from the gastro-intestinal tract generally allow efficient uptake, there are important differences in the absorption rates for different oils[46] and these differences may be reflected in the apparent acute toxicology of chemicals tested in this way.

Some ingested particulates may be absorbed from the lumen of the intestines[27]. Chemicals with molecular radii of less than 4 nm may be absorbed directly through pores in the lining membrane and this direct uptake is called 'convective absorption'. As with the stomach, the contents of the intestines influence toxicant absorption and the following factors may modify toxicant uptake at locations throughout the whole gastro-intestinal tract.

(a) Influence of contents on digestive physiology at the cellular level[37,47-50]
(b) Influence of contents on gastric emptying and/or intestinal mobility[35-38,50]
(c) Influence on the formation of complexes between the toxicant and

intestinal contents thus facilitating or diminishing the rate of uptake of the toxicant[34,51]

Toxification, as well as destruction and detoxification, can occur within the alimentary tract and these metabolic effects may be associated with the intrinsic physiological function of the alimentary tract or may be due to the microflora present within the tract[52]. For example, there are marked species differences in the acute toxicity of zinc phosphide, these differences are reflected in the pattern of release of gastric hydrochloric acid in different species, the acute toxicity of zinc phosphide being associated with the formation and subsequent absorption of phosphine[53].

$$Zn_3P_2 + 6 HCl \rightarrow 3 ZnCl_2 + 2 PH_3$$

Many products cause irritation of the gastro-intestinal tract and this irritation may directly influence absorption or, in some cases, the irritation may indirectly influence acute toxicity by causing vomitting. In predictive acute toxicity testing the administration of excessive volumes of toxicants by gavage is both irresponsible and scientifically indefensible as the physical distribution of the product will affect meaningful observations. It has been recommended that for the laboratory rat, five millilitres of any liquid per one kilogram of body weight (5 ml kg^{-1}), by gavage, should not be exceeded and it is imperative that similar limitations should be applied to the volume of toxicant administered by gavage to any other species used for investigative purposes.

Absorption of some chemicals from the rectum can be very efficient and the possibility of adverse effects of drugs administered by this route must not be neglected. The anal submucosa of many species contain a network of inter-connecting veins and the blood from this network is conveyed, by means of the superior rectal vein, into the portal vein or through the middle and inferior rectal veins which feed directly into the systemic system thus by-passing the liver; hence, in these species, toxicants absorbed via the rectum do not wholly pass through the hepatic metabolizing system[25,54-56]. Species differences are important in investigative toxicology and this route is no exception. Rectal absorption in the rat is associated entirely with the systemic circulation[56], and it is known that even in species with the distribution split between portal and systemic, such as man, the actual distribution will be influenced by the physico-chemical nature of the absorbed toxicant[25].

For obvious reasons acute intoxication via the rectal route is uncommon with chemicals other than some classes of drugs. One example of a drug that has caused acute intoxication and death by this route is tribromoethanol when it has been used as a rectally administered anaesthetic in humans with hepatic insufficiency.

2.2.2 Intake via the respiratory tract (inhalation exposure)

Products can be inhaled as gases, vapours, droplets or particulates and the physical form of any inhaled substance can profoundly affect its potential for exerting acute toxic effects[57].

In order to understand inhalation toxicology a reasonable knowledge of the

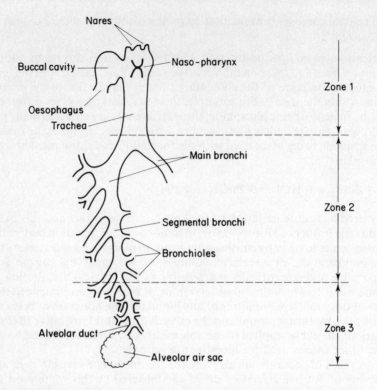

Fig. 2.5   Diagram of mammalian respiratory tree in relation to inhalation of toxicants.

anatomy and physiology of the respiratory system must be assumed and standard texts on the subject should be consulted by any reader unfamilar with the subject. Here it will suffice to consider a highly simplified representation of the typical mammalian respiratory tract (see Figure 2.5) which can be seen to have been divided into three zones. These three zones are not formal anatomic divisions but merely convenient delineations of the regions associated with uptake of toxicants[64].

Inhaled toxicants may enter the respiratory tract via the external nares (nostrils) or through the mouth. There is a close physical association between the respiratory tract and the buccal cavity; this anatomical proximity is of importance in relation to aspiration toxicity[4] as well as straightforward inhalation toxicology. Within Zone 1 air flow varies between laminar and turbulent and this air flow can be affected by some inhaled chemicals[634]. Irritants in particular can markedly alter the form of the air flow[58] and this can create an awareness of irritancy which may be a safeguard when there is a risk of chemicals being inhaled[633]. The potential protective value of irritancy is associated with the exposed subject being able to respond to the situation by diminishing the level of exposure but where there is no possibility of avoidance the irritation may be a significant aspect of the toxic response. Pulmonary oedema resulting from direct irritation is sometimes the prime cause of death associated with some volatile or gaseous toxicants (e.g. chlorine). Only a limited amount of toxicant absorption occurs in Zone 1. This region is associated more with a sieving effect on inhaled particulates and droplets than with absorption[59-61,618,634]. The absorptive characteristics of Zone 1 vary between species and this must be taken into account in predictive inhalation toxicology[664]. Zone 2 is predominantly concerned with air flow and only a little absorption occurs within this region. Droplets and particulates of intermediate size may be deposited within this zone[62,634].

Maximum absorption of inhaled toxicants occurs in Zone 3. This is the zone in which physiological gaseous interchanges occur between the inhaled atmosphere and the blood[618,633]. The surface area available for gaseous interchange is very large (e.g. in man this surface is estimated to be between 30 m^2 and 100 m^2). The lining of the alveoli consists of a thin moist epithelium which is readily penetrated by many chemicals. With gases and vapours it is sometimes assumed that the critical factor for absorption is the blood/air partition coefficient[63] but detailed studies of the absorption of several chemicals from the lungs of rats has indicated that the toxicokinetics are actually more complicated and that there are other factors involved in addition to the partition coefficient[64]. The lining epithelium of the lungs is readily penetrated by many organic solutes and penetration can be very rapid[65,618]. Once inhaled, lipid-insoluble solutes are far more efficiently absorbed from the lungs than from the alimentary tract[66]. Although there are exceptions, a high lipid/water partition coefficient generally favours uptake within the lungs but with both lipid-soluble and lipid-insoluble chemicals the penetration rate is directly related to the concentration of the chemical that is in contact with the lining epithelium. Toxicants in the form of gases or vapours enter the lungs mixed with air so that the concentration of toxicant in the inhaled atmosphere, duration of the exposure and the blood/air partition coefficient of the toxicant all govern the amount of toxicant that is absorbed. If an inhaled gas or vapour exhibits an irritant effect this can influence uptake within Zone 3 because of the damage to the epithelial lining[633].

In relation to inhalation toxicology, droplets and particulates are more complex in their behaviour than gases and vapours[634]. The movement characteristics of droplets and particles affects their uptake from the respiratory tract and their dynamic activities are very different from the static measurements associated with identical particles and droplets[67]. Some of the most important characteristics of droplets and particles, in relation to inhalation toxicology, are shown in Table 2.1. Research has been carried out to define the distribution characteristics of particles and droplets within the respiratory tract and some very precise measurements have been made[68,69]. It is clear from Table 2.1 that the physical characteristics of inhaled materials will affect distribution within the respiratory tract and to this must be added the effects of the respiratory rate and the tidal volume[70,71] and also the anatomy of the respiratory tract of the exposed species[72]. Even within a species there can be substantial physiological differences[73,74] and the magnitude of these differences between individuals can be problematic to any investigator who has to design, perform or interpret predictive acute inhalation toxicity tests[75,635].

The fundamental similarities of the processes associated with the inhalation of toxicants and some of the situations associated with chemical engineering has given impetus to the search for expression of the toxicodynamics of inhalation

Table 2.1   Some physical factors that may influence the deposition of particles and droplets in the respiratory tract.

Characteristic	Comments
Particle size or droplet size	(a) Atmospheres, however generated, always contain an array of different sizes of particles or droplets. (b) Particle and droplet size must be considered in terms of aerodynamic diameters and not static measurements.
Inertia	When the air-stream changes direction within the respiratory tract inertia may not permit the particles to change direction and deposition may occur
Gravity	If air-stream movement is small then gravity can cause precipitation of particles or droplets.
Brownian movement	Bombardment of particles or droplets by air molecules can create a state of Brownian movement within the alveoli.
Aggregation or coagulation of particles or droplets	Larger particles or droplets are more easily deposited than small ones.
Condensation with water	Uptake of water by droplets or particles increases size and encourages deposition.
Thermal conductivity	If thermal conductivity of the particle or droplet is low then the warmth of the lung wall repels towards the lumen and the air-stream carries away.
Electric charge	Charge on the particle or droplet relative to charge on wall of tract will either encourage or discourage deposition.

exposure in terms of mathematical models[71,76], and this approach may yet prove to be helpful in refining the techniques of predictive inhalation toxicology[69-74,635].

There are some corollaries between inhalation toxicology and the respiratory uptake of toxicants from water by aquatic dwelling vertebrate animals (i.e. fish and some amphibians) although there are major differences between terrestial and aquatic vertebrates in terms of the respiratory tract anatomy and also in the physiology of respiration.

2.2.3 Intake by percutaneous and perocular absorption

The skin, together with its appendages, and the eyes effectively comprise the outer surface of the vertebrate animal. Contact between the external surfaces of the body and potential toxicants occurs frequently and contact may result from deliberate, accidental or adventitious exposure.

Although the skin possesses selective barrier properties many chemicals are able to penetrate the barrier and, once absorbed, systemic effects occur.

The skin is not a homogeneous organ with the physical characteristics of a uniform membrane. Some of the ways in which skin differs from a simple membrane are associated with the following facts:

(a) Skin is a dynamic living organ[77].

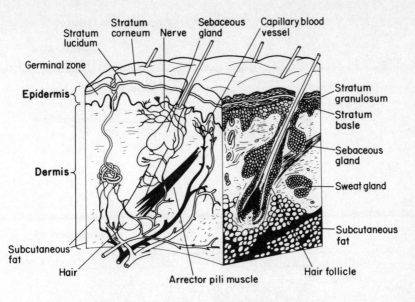

Fig. 2.6 A diagrammatic three-dimensional section of mammalian skin.

(b) Skin is capable of metabolic activity albeit the processes are slower than comparable processes in most other organs[78].

(c) Skin is not a homogeneous structure and there are important differences associated with different anatomic locations within any individual (e.g. thickness of epidermis, presence or absence of sweat glands, follicles, etc.)[79].

(d) No two species have identical skins although the basic anatomy may have characteristics in common[80,81].

Within the limitations of (c) and (d) above, Figures 2.6 and 2.7 are diagrammatic representations of typical structures of the skin found in the majority of mammalian species (n.b. the skins of non-mammalian species differ from those shown in Figures 2.6 and 2.7). Penetration of chemicals through mammalian skin (i.e. percutaneous absorption) occurs either by passage through the epidermis, using either intracellular or intercellular routes, or by passage via one or more of the physiological sub-structures (i.e. sebaceous apparatus or sweat glands). Transepidermal absorption is the principal percutaneous route of entry for toxicants[82] but the hair follicles, sebaceous glands and, occasionally, sweat glands can be important in the translocation of some toxicants[83].

From time to time it has been suggested that there might be a specific barrier zone within the skin. Although this was recognized by Szakall[624] its existence has sometimes been doubted; more recently, Bowser and co-workers[623] have reported on their research into epidermal permeability and concluded that the barrier function of the epidermis is associated with a hydroxylated linoleate derivative which may be formed in the lower stratum corneum region. More research will be required before the full story of the percutaneous penetration phenomenon is understood.

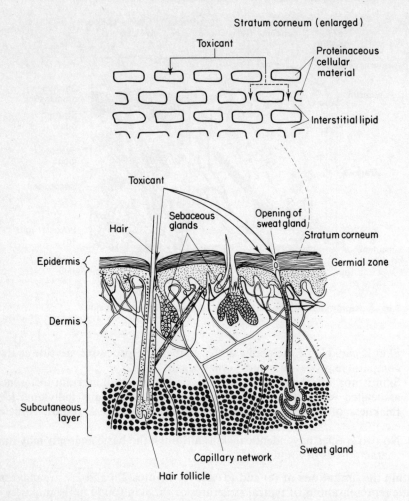

Fig. 2.7   A diagrammatic cross-section of mammalian skin. Most toxicants penetrate through the stratum corneum (inter- and intra-cellular routes), some lipid-soluble toxicants may penetrate via the sebaceous glands and a small amount (generally negligible) of hydrophilic toxicants may penetrate via sweat glands.

Some chemicals readily penetrate the skin whereas others only penetrate it with difficulty[22]. The major characteristics of a toxicant that affect its ability to penetrate mammalian skin are shown in Table 2.2 and the main characteristics of skin that influence penetrability by toxicants are listed in Table 2.3.

Once any toxicant has penetrated through the epidermis the dynamics of uptake by the vasculature becomes very important[84] and this, in turn, may be influenced by the effects of the toxicant *per se*, or its vehicle, on the vasculature (i.e. vasodilatation or vasoconstriction influence the rate of uptake and hence toxic response[85]). In respect of both acute and sub-acute toxicology, the rate of percutaneous penetration is critical to the response.

Skin is not a simple membrane but some models of the percutaneous

Table 2.2 Some characteristics of toxicants that influence ability to penetrate skin

Characteristic	Comments
Ionic state	Undissociated molecules penetrate better than ions but some ionized chemicals can penetrate.
Molecular size	Small molecules penetrate better than large molecules but some macromolecules can penetrate skin.
Lipophilicity	Lipophilicity favours skin penetration but some water soluble chemicals can penetrate skin.
Viscosity	Increasing viscosity diminishes skin penetrability.
Concentration of toxicant	Skin penetration is affected by the concentration of toxicant.
Facilitation	The penetrability characteristics of a toxicant can be affected by the vehicle in which it is formulated; the penetrability may be increased or reduced.

penetration characteristics of chemicals have been developed on the basis of membrane physics[86,87,621]; and some useful *in vitro* data have been obtained by using isolated skin, in appropriate diffusion cells[88]. Skin penetration characteristics have been linked to modifications of Fick's Law of Diffusion[89-91]; but caution is always necessary with extrapolation of these data to the *in vivo* situation[621].

On the basis of a perceived need to assess the most unfavourable toxic rating it has been a long established practice in predictive toxicology to use contact between the toxicant and the skin under an occlusive dressing[92,93]. The materials used for the occlusive covering can be very important[93] and it is necessary to be aware that volatile chemicals and also products that damage skin will both

Table 2.3 Some characteristics of skin that influence penetrability by toxicants

Characteristic	Comments
Species	Skins of different species differ greatly in their penetrability.
Anatomical location	Skin varies in its penetrability characteristics in different locations on the same animal.
Health and skin damage	Many dermatological conditions can affect penetrability.
Hydration of skin	Water content of the stratum corneum affects penetration.
Ambient temperature	Skin penetrability can be altered by raising or lowering the ambient temperature.
Occlusion	Absorption of toxicants is generally more efficient if the exposure occurs under an occlusive covering.
Vehicle effects	Some solvents, or other components of vehicles used to formulate toxicants, can increase or decrease the skin penetration characteristics by direct tissue damage or degreasing effect.

appear to be substantially more toxic when contact is under an occlusive covering than if the surface is exposed.

It is difficult to visualize that any chemical could be less toxic when applied under an occlusive dressing than when contact is with uncovered skin and certainly occlusion promotes the formation of toxicant reservoirs in the skin and this, in turn, leads to a more prolonged uptake[87].

The eyes are partially protected from exposure to chemicals by various physiological means such as the blink reflex and surface flushing of the eyes with tears. In addition to the physiological protection, humans but not other species, exhibit strong psychological associations with ocular damage and thus may be persuaded to take additional protective action (i.e. use of physical barriers such as goggles, visors, etc.) but, even so, accidental and adventitious ocular exposures sometimes occur. Deliberate ocular contact with chemicals is not uncommon (e.g. some drugs and cosmetics are applied to the eyes) and, absorption may result in systemic intoxication.

The small surface area of eyes, coupled with the protective physiological mechanisms, makes the chances of systemic intoxication by the perocular route considerably less than by other exposure routes. Once contact has occurred, perocular penetration is dependent on the degree of ionization of the toxicants involved and on their lipid-solubility[94,95]. Plumbism has been observed in women from the Indian sub-continent using eye cosmetics containing lead salts. Systemic intoxication has been observed in some patients undergoing treatment with potent anticholinesterase agents applied to the eye in the form of drops[96] and, in the laboratory, sometimes products induce signs of systemic intoxication during routine testing for eye irritation potential and this symptomatology must not be disregarded by the investigator.

2.2.4 Intake by parenteral exposure

By convention, the term **parenteral exposure** is restricted to include only administration of toxicants by injection whereas semantically parenteral should include all routes other than those involving the alimentary tract. If it was not for this convention, parenteral exposure would include the inhalation, percutaneous and perocular routes but these three routes are excluded.

In order to describe routes of injection the organ or tissue involved is prefaced by either **intra-** (meaning into) or **sub-** (meaning below). Thus an injection into the musculature is termed an intramuscular injection whereas a subcutaneous injection is one in which the chemical is injected into the tissue immediately below the skin.

In predictive acute toxicology it may be necessary to mimic the parenteral routes to be used for therapeutic agents or sometimes parenteral routes are utilized to obtain information relating to the toxicokinetics of the product although the route used may have little direct relevance to likely exposure[97].

The intraperitoneal route is commonly used for the administration of chemicals in experimental toxicology but this route of administration is rarely used in therapeutics because of the substantial risk of peritonitis and other traumas; also it can be a painful procedure.

The surface area of the membrane lining the peritoneal cavity is very large and allows rapid absorption of many types of chemical; the absorption of some chemicals from the peritoneal cavity is so rapid that the resultant effects may closely mimic those associated with intravenous injection of the toxicant. For practical purposes the peritoneum can be considered as having two distinct parts: One part envelops most of the abdominal organs (visceral peritoneum) and the other lines the walls of the abdomen (parietal peritoneum). Those chemicals that are absorbed by the visceral peritoneum drain into the portal venous system and thence pass to the liver where toxification or detoxification may occur. A smaller quantity of the chemical will be absorbed via the parietal peritoneum and drain directly into the systemic circulation thus by-passing the liver[98]. Although absorption from the peritoneal cavity is generally rapid, uptake is not always linear with time[99]. The peritoneum is very sensitive to the effects of irritants and the irritant properties of a chemical administered by this route can affect uptake and can cause suffering to the recipient; the implications of this must not be disregarded by any investigator utilizing this route of exposure.

There are three main reasons for the popularity of the intraperitoneal route in investigative toxicology: (a) it is technically easier to use than the intravenous route, (b) it is possible to use solutions of toxicants in oils for intraperitoneal but not intravenous injection, and (c) by using intraperitoneal injection for investigative purposes the vagaries of metabolic change that are associated with the alimentary tract are avoided.

If products under investigation are administered by either the intramuscular or subcutaneous routes then slow rates of uptake will be experienced. These two routes are often used for drugs in therapeutics in order to prolong effects and the kinetics of absorption from the subcutaneous and intramuscular routes have been extensively investigated in relation to therapeutic pharmacokinetics[100-107,682].

Parenteral administration by the subcutaneous and intramuscular route allows absorption from aqueous and from oily solutions and it is also possible to achieve absorption from suspensions of low solubility chemicals provided that the particle size is small enough. A large proportion of any chemical administered by either the subcutaneous or the intramuscular route will not pass through the liver before circulating to targets in the body.

Toxicokinetics associated with intramuscular injection varies with the site of injection. For example, when the drug diazepam is injected into the deltoid its potency almost equates to that following oral administration whereas injection into the gluteus only allows a slow uptake of the drug.

The most rapid means for a toxicant to enter into the circulation is by direct injection into the blood-stream and this is achieved by intravenous injection and occasionally by intra-arterial injection. Following either intravenous or intra-arterial injection the distribution of the toxicant to the target sites is rapid and the liver is mainly by-passed[97] but there can be quantitative variation in the response depending on which artery or vein is used for the injection[108].

Caution is necessary when either the intravenous or the intra-arterial routes are being investigated for many chemicals will damage the blood vessels and some may react with components of the blood. Chemicals that are immiscible with blood (e.g. oils) cannot be administered directly into the blood-stream without the risk of embolism. Similarly any chemicals of formulations that form a precipitate on dilution with blood are likely to require an alternative route for administration (e.g. intraperitoneal injection).

If the product to be administered is water miscible and non-irritant to the vasculature, there remain three factors to be taken into account:

(a) **Tonicity**
Ideally any product injected into the blood-stream should be isotonic with the cellular components of the blood. Hypertonic and hypotonic injections affect some of the erythrocytes and other cells, particularly those located near the site of the injection, but once the injection has been achieved dilution by the blood will tend to diminish the osmotic effect.

(b) **Time**
The speed with which the toxicant is injected into the blood-stream can influence the toxicological response. Rapid injection into the blood-stream can prove far more acutely toxic than when the same quantity of the toxicant is administered slowly; for this reason it is essential in toxicology that the rate of injection is defined and controlled.

(c) **Temperature**
Ideally products injected into the blood-stream should be at approximately body temperature when administered; both heat and cold can influence response. Some chemicals react with blood causing an exothermic reaction and this may be unacceptable.

Specialized investigations in toxicology sometimes require products to be injected directly into organs and tissues of the central nervous system. Technically these injections require skill and great care[109] and their use tends to be associated with the need to study direct effects of molecules on parts of the central nervous system without the influence of *in vivo* metabolism[110] and also avoidance of other factors associated with the distribution of chemicals into cerebrospinal fluid and translocation across the blood–brain barrier[111,112].

Techniques for continuous parenteral administration of drugs are becoming important in therapeutics. There can be little doubt that these techniques will find an important place in the design of sub-acute toxicity tests but, as yet, there is a long way to go before this technology becomes commonplace in laboratories. Sub-acute parenteral toxicology obviously necessitates multiple injections and great care must be taken to avoid the trauma of local tissue damage.

2.3 Formulation Effects

Whereas every chemical has a potential for causing toxic effects, the way in which any product is presented to the target can substantially alter its acute toxic potential. Formulation can change the pattern of toxicokinetics and may increase or decrease the apparent toxicity of the individual ingredients. Any components used in the formulation of a product will have toxicity potentials of their own and sometimes the toxicities of these ingredients may be intrinsically important in relation to the acute toxicity of the total formulation. Often the toxic effects of formulations are brought about by acceleration, or a retardation, of uptake of the most toxic ingredient. The influence of ingredients on the toxicity of any formulation will differ considerably depending on route of exposure. The influence of formulation on toxicity, as well as effects on efficacy, is of great importance when considering the presentation of chemicals for use[26]. Formulation effects are deliberatively developed in the presentation of therapeutic agents or pesticides and must not be disregarded when risk/benefit analyses are being considered[586].

It is common practice to express the acute toxicity of a formulation in terms of the amount of active ingredient producing the toxic effect although it would be more meaningful to express the exposure as an amount of the whole formulation. This practice is complicated by the fact that there is not a simple relationship between amount of toxicant in a formulation and its acute toxicity rating: for some products, and for some routes of exposure, an increase in the concentration of the toxicant in a formulation will increase its toxicity rating whereas for some other chemicals it is decreasing the concentration that increases the toxicity rating[113-116].

In investigative acute toxicology there is a logistic problem associated with the effects of concentration on acute toxicity rating. It is often arbitrary whether the product being investigated is administered in a series of amounts that are based on a single formulation with the volumes that are administered being varied (i.e. the concentration of toxicant in the vehicle remains fixed), or, whether a series of different concentrations of the toxicant are used and the volume administered is kept constant. Both of these methods are commonly used by investigators and may give rise to different acute toxicity ratings for the same toxicant. It can be argued that where the investigation relates to the acute toxicity of a liquid product then it is not logical to introduce concentration effects by dilution with a vehicle and that tests using variable volumes of undiluted material are the best criteria of acute toxicity. For products that have to be diluted for administration (e.g. solids) the choice of dosing method is arbitrary. The method of administration, whether using constant concentration or constant volume, should be documented for the acute toxicity rating of products.

The selection of vehicles that may be used for toxicity testing requires care. Apart from any influence that the vehicle may exert on the uptake and distribution of the toxicant there is the added possibility of chemical interaction between toxicants and vehicles and checking for compatibility is essential.

Some products can be administered undiluted thus obviating the need for a vehicle. For peroral administration it is sometimes practicable to encapsulate the toxicant in gelatin, or some similar material, but this involves filling each capsule on an individual animal basis in order to achieve the correct dose per body weight and this can be a labour intensive procedure if large numbers of test animals are to be exposed to the product. Capsules may be used for solids or liquids provided that the gelatin, or other material, does not react with the toxicant. Techniques are available for the administration of capsules to most species used in laboratory investigations[117-120] but the toxicant does not come into contact with the buccal cavity (see section 2.2) and is not released in the alimentary tract until the capsule has been digested by the gastric contents.

The same criteria apply to the methodology for sub-acute toxicity testing as have been described for acute testing. Some products can be administered in sub-acute regimens in undiluted form whereas others need formulation to facilitate administration.

The fact that apparently innocuous vehicles may exert important effects on the toxicology of a compound is often overlooked or disregarded by investigators. For example, corn oil is commonly regarded as a bland solvent and yet it is known that when carbon tetrachloride is administered by intra-gastric gavage in corn oil its hepatotoxicity is enhanced[676].

As an alternative to the use of vehicles for the administration of toxicants by the oral route, it is sometimes convenient to administer toxicants in capsule form. Sub-acute investigations are often carried out with the toxicant administered in admixture with diet or dissolved in the drinking water. If the toxicant is being administered in either of these ways it is essential to know the stability of the toxicant under the test conditions. Quite apart from the possibility of interactions occurring between food components, or water and the added toxicant there is also the possibility of loss due to volatility or adsorption onto container surfaces. These are practical problems and examples are helpful. Volatile chemicals (e.g. solvents, some pesticides, etc.) may have a short concentration stability (i.e. the concentration half-life may be only minutes or hours) because of loss to the atmosphere from the diet; certainly some of the earlier investigations of the sub-acute toxicology of such chemicals were not adequately monitored for this possibility and the reported findings for the studies, based on nominal exposure levels, must be viewed with caution. Some chemicals are strongly adsorbed onto surfaces; for example, some of the pyrethroid insecticides can be removed from water by adsorption onto the container surface. Actual chemical interactions between added toxicant and components of the food are not uncommon and may lead to the findings of the investigation being associated with by-products rather than the parent compound. Ethylene oxide, used for fumigation, reacts with chloride ions in foodstuff to form ethylenechlorohydrin[679], early studies on the toxicology of ethylene oxide in diet were carried out on the basis of nominal ethylene oxide concentration but in the ignorance of the implications of the relatively large amounts of ethylenechlorohydrin that were present.

Both in acute and sub-acute predictive testing, investigators must be alert to the possibility of unexpected interference. To illustrate this two examples have been chosen, both of these have been known to occur in laboratories with highly competent investigators. Firstly, if a suspension of a solid toxicant in a vehicle is forced, under pressure, along a tube (i.e. an intraoesophageal dosing catheter or an hypodermic needle) there will be a filtering effect, this leads to a build-up of the solid component inside the tube while the liquid vehicle, with a diminished amount of solid component, is expelled, hence a smaller amount of solid component is actually received by the animal despite the correct dose having been chosen and put into the syringe. A note of caution is pertinent here, for not only will the test be invalid but there is a physical hazard, namely that the filtering effect leads to back pressure in the equipment and this may cause the dosing catheter, or needle, to separate from the syringe thus allowing toxicant to be sprayed over the surrounding area. Secondly, chemical interactions sometimes occur between toxicants and the materials used to fabricate equipment (e.g. solvents attacking plastics, acids interacting with metals, etc.). It may be necessary to investigate this possibility before commencing on the toxicity test. The composition of laboratory animals diets may influence the toxicity of some chemicals[393,668,669] and this may not be obvious at the outset of any investigation. Investigators may have to be prepared to carry out several modified studies in order to even locate this type of effect since it may not be obvious from the results of one investigation. Investigations into the sub-acute inhalation toxicology of chemicals are fraught with the problems of gaseous adsorption onto the surfaces of chamber walls, electrostatic precipitation of particulates and various other physico–chemical phenomena. Meaningful inhalation studies require adequate knowledge of physical chemistry and should not be undertaken without appropriate expertise being available[635,636].

2.4 Other Physical Factors

Responses to acute exposures can be influenced by numerous physical factors. Some of the most important factors are detailed below.

2.4.1 Duration of exposure

Duration of exposure can be of critical importance in acute toxicology and yet it may be difficult to define time-span with a precise meaning in this context. To illustrate this point consider a simple one target receptor model (Figure 2.8): the time for the toxicant to enter the organism (t_1) will be influenced by the nature of the exposure; it may be rapid (e.g. as with intravenous injection) or it may be slow (e.g. as with a lipophobic toxicant penetrating the skin). Intake time (t_1) will be offset, at least in part, by the breakdown and excretion rates (t_4) for the toxicant in the particular target species and this may be so efficient that insufficient amounts of the toxicant molecules reach the critical receptors within the organism[121]. If it is assumed that some of the toxicant molecules reach the receptor site in time t_2 it will be necessary for critical levels to be achieved and

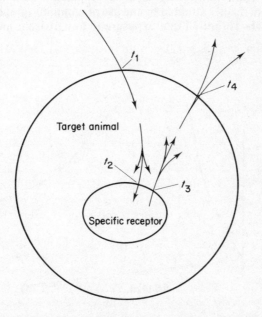

Fig. 2.8 A simple model in which the toxicant–target interaction is limited to one specific receptor with toxicokinetic times shown as t_1, t_2, t_3, and t_4.

this has to be offset by the time (t_3) needed for removal of the toxicant molecules from the receptor[122,123]. Whereas in therapeutics the balance of t_1 and t_2 with t_3 and t_4 is carefully maintained in order to produce the desired effect, acute toxicology is more often associated with situations in which the overall system is flooded with excesses of the toxicant molecules and this balance is perturbed[121-123].

In predictive acute toxicology the total swamping of receptor systems by excessive exposures may kill animals whilst leaving the investigator unable to attribute a specific cause of death[123]. In order to overcome this problem it is sometimes necessary to undertake further detailed investigations but using sub-lethal exposures to reveal details of the mode of action of the toxicant; this is a major purpose of sub-acute toxicity testing.

Clearly the simple model discussed above, and illustrated in Figure 2.8, does not take into acount the situation that occurs when it is not the parent molecule that influences the receptor. When the effect is due to one or more metabolites being formed within the organism (i.e. toxification), it is the metabolite or metabolites that act at the receptor site. In this situation it is necessary to consider the time for conversion of the parent molecule to metabolites and then the time for the metabolite to influence the receptor.

For some situations the exposure time (t_1) may take the form of a continuum rather than an instantaneous, one-off, event. This continuum is very apparent with inhalation exposures and it also occurs as a result of contamination of the skin by a toxicant. In these situations it is necessary to relate the exposure to its duration as well as to the total quantity of toxicant. The relationship between quantity of toxicant, duration of exposure and response can be illustrated conveniently by means of three-dimensional graphical presentations (see Figure 2.9) and these are readily attained by the use of computer-graphics[617].

It must never be forgotten that exposure to any toxicant may influence the

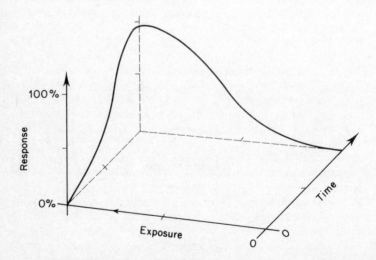

Fig. 2.9 A typical three-dimensional graph relating response to exposure (dose) and time. Families of curves can be achieved for variations in any of the three parameters.

ongoing toxicokinetics and thus the pattern of events, at least quantitatively, may vary with duration of exposure[637]. This can be a contributory factor to the development of tolerance in toxicological response[638]. The rule that is attributed to Häber[124] states that the multiple of concentration (dose) and time of exposure (duration) is directly related to response. Häber's Rule is known to be only approximately correct but, used with care, it can, occasionally provide useful information[125]. Although Häber's Rule[124] is most commonly utilized in relation to inhalation exposure and ecotoxicology (e.g. aquatic exposure toxicology), it is sometimes applied as a simple guide-line for the choice of exposure levels for long-term and chronic toxicity testing when the only available data on which the selection of exposure levels can be made is the findings from acute and sub-acute investigations; although this is a legitimate experimental ploy, it is not meaningful to assume that long-term or chronic studies can be replaced by the simple expedient of applying Häber's Rule to the results of sub-acute tests. Utilization of time interval between exposure and death (i.e. a composite of t_1, t_2, t_3, and t_4 when death is the defined end-point of the toxic response) in the same way that the lethal dose is often used as an expression of acute toxicity rating has been explored [126]. The formal relationship between estimated lethal time may vary from the actual time to death, or in alternative terms, the survival time: this apparent anomaly is attributable to statistical variation of the data from symmetry[126]. Survival time does not have wide application in predictive acute toxicology[126].

Many predictive sub-acute toxicity tests are designed so that a constant amount of toxicant is administerd daily to animals. Many sub-acute exposures are like this in practice. If the rate of elimination of the toxicant from the body of the target is at a constant rate and the elimination follows first-order kinetics, then the quantity of toxicant remaining in the body rises towards a constant level (i.e. the tissue level's plateau). The time taken to reach the plateau level is a function of the half-life of the toxicant in the target.

The maximum concentration of the toxicant in the tissues will occur at some time after exposure and this will be dependent on the rate of absorption. If, as is the case with most toxicants, the rate of elimination is not so fast that total elimination occurs before the next exposure, then the level in the body of the target will build-up until the plateau is reached (see Figure 2.10). Clearly the exposure interval is critical to the findings for any particular toxicant and this raises the important issue in predictive toxicity testing, in other words, it is essential to standardize the exposure interval used in any investigation and it is not sensible to design experiments that involve daily dosing on working weekdays but not on holidays (e.g. weekends) and then start up again after the break.

The principle of body burden plateauing does not apply to all toxicants[663]. If the toxicant is removed from the body by a saturable mechanism there must be a maximum rate for the elimination pathway and hence elimination cannot increase indefinitely to cope with the increasing amount of toxicant in the body, this leads to accumulation of toxicant in the body. Cumulative toxicity occurs with many chemicals (e.g. heavy metals, polychlorinated biphenyls, etc.). Changes in the toxicokinetic capabilities of the body with age can be an important factor and must be taken into account when investigating sub-acute toxicology. In the therapeutics of inflammatory conditions this has become very apparent; because of changes in the elimination half-lives of some of the non-

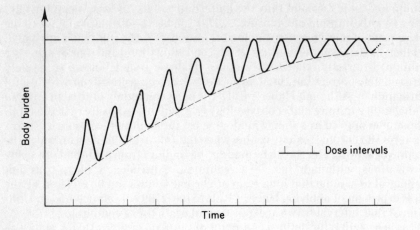

Fig. 2.10   Diagrammatic representation of plateau effect resulting from exposure to a constant amount of toxicant at regular intervals and assuming that elimination follows first order kinetics.

steroidal anti-inflammatory drugs in elderly patients there has been toxic sequalae in some people treated with dose levels that are quite acceptable in younger patients[647]. Conversely, human adults are able to conjugate ingested salicylates with glycine to facilitate elimination from the body whereas human infants are unable to conjugate salicylates in this way, or at least only slowly, and show poor tolerance to this group of chemicals.

Obviously between species differences in toxicokinetics will influence the validity of predictive sub-acute toxicity tests. Ideally no sub-acute study is carried out without a thorough consideration of comparative toxicokinetics.

2.4.2 Bioavailability of the toxicants

The acute toxicity potential of any product is influenced by its bio-availability[127-135] and some of the most important criteria of bioavailability are considered here:

(a) Particle size

Generally it may be anticipated that the greater the surface area of any particulate material then the more absorption will be facilitated. This generalization applies to all routes of exposure[136,137] but has to be related to the physical interaction with gas movement within the respiratory tract during and following respiratory exposure[70]. Detailed definition of particulate size characteristics is essential for any predictive acute toxicity testing carried out with solid materials and this physical definition must not be omitted from investigations involving suspensions of solids for peroral or parenteral exposures. The toxicokinetics of encapsulated solids administered by the alimentary route and the uptake of solid materials that are in contact with skin are both influenced by particle size.

Information on physical characteristics is needed in relation to therapeutic actions of drugs, interpretation of dust effects in industrial hygiene and also for the optimization of pesticidal activity. Data obtained for these purposes may also provide useful information on particulate characteristics relating to their acute toxicology.

(b) Viscosity

By all routes of exposure an increase in viscosity is associated with diminished absorbability and conversely decreases in viscosity facilitate absorption[138,139]. Viscosity influences toxicokinetics in the alimentary tract by modifying gastro-intestinal transit rate and also by altering the ability of the toxicant to make contact with the absorptive surface[26,139].

Particle size [see (a) above] can influence the viscosity of materials. It is common practice in the formulation of chemicals that are insoluble in water to use suspending agents to aid dispersion and this is often achieved by means of suspending agents such as vegetable gums (e.g. acacia, tragacanth, etc.) or carboxymethylcellulose. The viscosity of the formulation is influenced by the amount of suspending agent used, the concentration and particle size of the suspended ingredient and the temperature of the suspension[137,140-142].

There can be physico–chemical interaction between toxicants and suspending agents and the dissolution rate may be changed with a consequent influence on the acute toxicity of the product.

(c) Surfactant effects

Surfactants are sometimes included in formulations in order to improve the suspension characteristics of insoluble components and, sometimes, to improve the wetting characteristics of the formulation (e.g. pesticides for foliar application). In general, surfactants facilitate absorption of toxicants within the gastro-intestinal tract[143] and also increase the possibility of skin penetration by toxicants following the exposure[91,144,145].

(d) Formulations for parenteral exposure

In pharmaceutical development care has to be exercised in the choice of vehicles to be used for the parenteral administration of drugs and similar constraints must be applied to the choice of vehicles used in any investigation of acute toxicity by parenteral routes. In addition to ensuring that there is no unacceptable interaction between toxicant and vehicle it is also necessary that vehicles do not cause tissue reactions at the location of injection. Some vehicles are useful for this purpose but the choice is dependent on the route of exposure[146-148]; for example, oily solutions of toxicants may be administered by intraperitoneal injection but not by intravenous injection (see Section 2.2.4).

What may appear to be minor differences in formulation can sometimes have marked effects on the acute toxicity of some products. To illustrate this point, it has been shown that paraquat can be administered to mice intravenously, either in the form of an aqueous solution or dissolved in physiological saline, and the responses to these two formulations are the same, however the presence of sodium chloride in a solution reduces the acute toxicity of paraquat to mice if it is administered by either the intraperitoneal or subcutaneous routes when the acute toxicity is compared with aqueous solutions administered in the same way[149]. The possibility that even seemingly trivial modifications in dosage form can markedly influence toxicokinetics must not be overlooked in the design and interpretation of acute and sub-acute toxicity tests.

3
Predictive Tests (*in vivo*)

Predictive acute and sub-acute toxicity testing are carried out with the objective of assessing the toxic potential of the test material, under conditions of either acute or sub-acute exposure, in one set of animals and then using the information derived from those animals to predict the toxic potential in other animals. Even if the animals used for the test are of the same type as the ones to which the data will be applied there will be individual differences in susceptibility. Most often toxicology is concerned with much bigger problems in extrapolation of data as the majority of predictive tests are carried out using animals that are very different from the target species of ultimate interest[290-293,296-314].

Predictive testing that is intended to provide information on the toxicity of chemicals to vertebrate pests (e.g. vermin) can sometimes be carried out using the species of ultimate interest or at least closely related species may be available for investigative purposes. For example, there is no reason why a rodenticide cannot be tested using various rodent species possibly including the specific vermin of ultimate concern. For many species there are constraints on their use in investigative toxicology. If man is the target species of most concern, as is often the case, then there are cogent ethical, moral and legal limitations on the use of man as an experimental test species and these limitations have been set out in the internationally accepted Declaration of Helsinki[150]. Quite apart from the ethical, moral and legal aspects, man is an extremely heterogeneous species and great care is necessary when interpretating results following human exposure.

For some products it is possible to obtain useful toxicological information from human experience without the need to perform predictive acute toxicity tests in other species[151]. Some of these data are acquired from professional monitoring of:

(i) accidentally or adventitiously exposed victims,
(ii) cases of deliberate misuse (e.g. suicides) and
(iii) controlled human experimentation with deliberate exposure to 'safe' levels of the product (i.e. as in clinical trials with new therapeutic agents).

Not all of the potentially available information from (i) and (ii) are obtained with the scientific rigour that is necessary for meaningful use by toxicologists but, none the less, there are signs of increasing professional awareness of the importance of comprehensive toxicological information[14]. The acquisition of toxicological data by using deliberately exposed humans requires a very high level of ethical awareness by any investigator. The dividing line between 'informed agreement' by the participants and undue risk may be blurred and the balance of the risk/benefit equation can all too easily be swayed by over enthusiasm; the motivation of people to participate for reward (e.g. prisoners seeking remission of sentence, students attracted by financial inducements, patients seeking miraculous cures, etc.) may tempt some investigators to take unnecessary risks and stringent precautions must be imposed to avoid this situation[150,295]. The deliberate use of involuntary human exposure, as for example happened in Nazi concentration camps, is contemplated with such total abhorrence by every toxicologist as to require no further elaboration or comment here.

When the target of ultimate concern is a species other than man then the choice of experimental model has to be based on known species characteristics. The avicidal and piscicidal properties of chemicals can be assessed in the laboratory using bird and fish species respectively but data obtained with birds in aviaries and fish in aquaria may differ from birds and fish in the wild[152,153]. Even in the wild there are very large differences in sensitivity exhibited by different species of birds and different species of fish to toxicants just as there are large differences between different mammalian species in their sensitivity to intoxication by some products[154].

The search for meaningful models in predictive acute toxicity testing is often subjugated to an absurd need for pseudo-respectable quantitative data rather than more meaningful, scientifically defensible, information[155]. In a different context it has been stated[156] that, 'It does require maturity to realize that models are to be used but not believed'. Every toxicologist concerned with predictive testing for acute and sub-acute effects must be prepared to apply rigorous scientific methodology in both the performance and the interpretation of these investigations if the models are to retain credibility.

3.1 Qualitative Aspects

Regrettably the term LD_{50} has become synonymous with acute toxicity testing in the minds of many people[163]. This misconception arises because of the frequency with which this convenient index, the LD_{50} value, has become the only way in which predictive acute toxicity data are presented. This approach must be eschewed if predictive acute toxicology is to become meaningful[163,574]. There are two particularly important aspects of acute intoxication that are not addressed by the LD_{50} value. These are the symptomatology and pathological changes occurring as a result of exposure but, with properly designed experiments, there is no reason why details of these can not be established during the assessment of the LD_{50} value[160,161]. Often, but not always, pathological changes are more readily discernible in sub-acute exposure experiments.

3.1.1 Symptomatology

Man is the only species capable of communicating subjective feelings to other people. No species, other than man, has this ability, hence if a toxicant causes subjective ill-feelings, for example, nausea and headache, only man can describe the sensation; there are no techniques for establishing whether an animal, other than man, is experiencing any sensations of adverse effect. Inability to recognize covert effects in experimental animals is a major shortcoming of *in vivo* predictive acute and sub-acute toxicity testing; in this respect the situation with *in vitro* methodology (see Chapter 4) is no better. These covert effects are called 'symptoms of intoxication' and, with humans, symptoms often provide an early warning that adverse effects are occurring.

Overt responses to exposure are called 'signs of intoxication' and these are not restricted to the subjective feelings of the exposed animals. Typical signs of intoxication include such observable episodes as convulsions, locomotor incoordination, sweating, etc. Although signs of intoxication can often be determined by *in vivo* predictive acute toxicity tests, the possibility of inter-species variation in response must always be taken into account. Signs of intoxication cannot be revealed by *in vitro* tests for predicting acute toxicity (see Chapter 4).

Some effects associated with acute intoxication may require specialized tests for their detection. These tests can be included in predictive acute toxicity testing in the laboratory but variations between species may be important:

(i)   physiological (e.g. electrocardiography to detect cardiac arrhythmias)
(ii) biochemical (e.g. serum transaminases measured to detect incipient hepatotoxicity)
(iii) behavioural (e.g. monitoring of activity)

To illustrate the importance of signs and symptoms in acute toxicology it is convenient to consider the pattern of events when vertebrates are poisoned with organophosphorus anti-cholinesterase agents (Table 3.1). There is a lot of experience of human intoxication with this class of compound[157-159] and the symptoms have frequently been sufficient for remedial action to be initiated but these symptoms are not detectable in predictive acute toxicity tests carried out using laboratory animals.

No predictive acute or sub-acute toxicity test is adequate without careful observation of the symptomatology[161]. With the development of new therapeutic agents it is common practice for the investigators to combine pharmacological studies with the tests for acute toxicity[160], and whenever possible this same combined approach should be used for other types of products as it may help to reveal important toxic properties.

Table 3.1   Characteristics of the symptomatology of acute intoxication in vertebrate species with organophosphorus anticholinesterase agents.

Signs		Symptoms	
Overt	Revealed	Subjective	Behavioural
sweating	diminished cholinesterase	headache	diminished ability to
vomitting	activities	nausea	concentrate
salivation	cardiac arrhythmias	abdominal pain	diminished acuity
miosis	increased blood pressure	cramp	
dyspnea		blurred vision	
diarrhoea			
muscular fasciculations			
cyanosis			
locomotor effects			

3.1.2 Pathological changes

Morphological changes may result from acute exposure to some toxicants. Some of these morphological changes will be detectable by gross visual examination of the carcass of the exposed animal or they may be more subtle and require much more detailed histopathological investigation. If death occurs rapidly following exposure to a toxicant it is unlikely that much will be gained by histopathological examination but gross *post mortem* examination of the cadaver may reveal some information (e.g. signs of corrosive effects[625]). If death is delayed until at least several days after the exposure then histopathological examination of the organs and tissues may reveal important toxicant-related changes. Detailed histological examinations are expensive, because of the skilled effort required, thus in predictive acute toxicity testing the experimental protocol should be designed to obtain the maximum of useful information with the minimum number of detailed necropsies. There is little merit in detailed examination of every animal in a conventional LD_{50} test when the relevant information is attainable by necropsies of a select portion of the exposed animals. Histopathological examinations of animals exhibiting delayed or prolonged signs of intoxication are essential.

The same discretionary principles apply to the need for haematological and physiological chemistry investigations of exposed animals. Sometimes it can be more helpful to investigate histopathological, haematological and physiological chemistry changes in groups of animals that have been exposed to repeated sub-lethal doses of the toxicant rather than acutely exposed animals but this forms part of the sub-acute rather than the acute toxicity testing programme.

There may be important species differences in response to any toxicant and the design of any predictive toxicity investigation, and interpretation of the results, must take this possibility into account[316]. To illustrate this point, it is probable that the delayed neuropathy associated with acute exposure to some organophosphorus compounds would be missed if rodents only are used for predictive toxicology, whereas this effect occurs in exposed humans and is known to be detectable by the use of some other readily available non-rodent laboratory species (e.g. domestic fowl).

3.2 Quantitative Aspects

An eminent physicist, Lord Kelvin (1824–1907), is reputed to have stated that; 'When you measure what you are speaking about and express it in numbers you know something about it, but when you cannot measure it, when you cannot express it in numbers, your knowledge is of a meagre and unsatisfactory kind'. No thinking person quibbles with the need for quantification in the physical sciences but there is much more controversy about the importance of the role of quantification in the biological sciences; this controversy has become apparent in relation to acute toxicity testing[155]. Some of the main arguments for and against quantification in acute toxicology are:

In favour of quantification

(a) Quantification formalises the relationship between exposure and response.
(b) Numeric data is more easily visualized than qualitative information.

(c) Storage and communication of quantitative data is easier than qualitative information.

(d) Reproducibility of numerically expressed data can be validated more easily than qualitative results.

(e) Interactive effects are more easily detected and their magnitude established by means of quantitative data whereas qualitative information is often too subjective to allow certainty.

(f) Some information can only be derived from quantitative data (e.g. therapeutic indices; hazard ratings, etc.).

Against Quantification

(a) Unnecessarily large numbers of test animals may be used to obtain statistically acceptable data when adequate information is obtainable by using less animals in well designed investigations.

(b) Precise data may lead to false assumptions of accuracy in what is an essentially qualitative subject.

(c) Quantification is weighted towards assumptions of homogeneity of response whereas in acute toxicology the exceptional individual within a population may be very important.

Too often quantification is considered to be an ultimate objective in acute toxicology when really it is no more than a convenient method for facilitating the handling of results[155,161-163,574]. The widespread requirement for acute toxicity data in regulatory matters has given impetus to the perceived need for quantification as it is easier to classify products on the basis of indices of toxicity, generally the LD_{50} values, rather than on the basis of qualitative descriptions of effects even if the latter are more meaningful[164].

For the majority of products it is found that toxic response increases with increasing magnitude of exposure until a maximum response is reached. If the exposure to the toxicant is sufficiently small there may be no apparent response. This phenomenon is called 'graded response' and can be explained in terms of the amount of the toxicant reaching the receptor sites ranging from insufficient to trigger a response to receptor saturation.

With therapeutic agents graded effects are important and the distinction between the desired pharmacological response and toxicity may not always be very great, this relationship is defined in terms of therapeutic indices. It is important to realize that sometimes the toxic response may involve separate receptors from those implicated to achieve the desired pharmacological effects; the relative ease with which different receptors are triggered may be critical to the safety of a product[165,166]. Although one pharmacological system may predominate in the response of an animal to exposure to a chemical there is always the possibility that other receptors may also be affected[121-123].

Graded responses are important in acute toxicology but, partly because of the preoccupation with quantification, it is more usual to concentrate on the 'all-or-none' type of response (i.e. the response either occurs or it does not occur). The 'all-or-none' response is defined mathematically as being a quantal response[167-169]. Biometricians have established mathematical relationships between graded and quantal responses[170] but for most purposes, certainly in acute toxicology, they should be considered as being quite distinct.

Any effect that results from exposure of an animal to a product can be quantitatively related to the magnitude of the exposure. The units used to express both response and exposure can be chosen to best define the overall situation and may be referred to as being the 'effect dose' (abbreviated to *ED*). If the effect occurs, or does not occur, and is dependent on the magnitude of the exposure (i.e. quantal response) then it should be possible to find the critical dose level at which the response just occurs, or conversely just does not occur, and this could be termed the 'threshold exposure'. In reality the 'threshold exposure' is very difficult to measure. In theory, the 'threshold exposure' level would have to be determined for each individual animal, and this is clearly not possible, so that a compromise is achieved by using more easily measurable population effects.

Population effects are quantified by exposing groups of animals to defined amounts of the product and assessing the proportion of animals, at each exposure level, that exhibit, or do not exhibit, the particular effect. The conventional way of expressing this information is to use percentage notation for the proportion of animals exhibiting the effect and then to state this percentage as a numeric value after the symbol *ED*. Thus the exposure, or dose level, corresponding to a 50% response is written as ED_{50} and the 20% response as ED_{20} and so on. Using this nomenclature it is not necessary to display the percent symbol (%) as this is automatically implied.

Death is a perfect form of quantal response because an animal can only be either dead or alive. Death is an obvious sequelae to some forms of intoxication hence death has become a much used criterion of acute toxicity. This use of death has been established in the nomenclature by the convention of using effect-dose (*ED*) values modified to lethal dose (*LD*) values, when the effect is death. Population effects are measured in terms of the numbers of animals killed by particular exposure or dose levels of toxicant. These population effects are expressed as LD_x values when x is the estimated percentage of those succumbing at the particular exposure level. Hence the exposure corresponding to 50% mortality is referred to as the LD_{50} value. It is necessary to note a variant of the nomenclature associated with situations in which the exposure is dynamically related to intake from the total environment, this occurs in relation to inhalation exposure and in aquatic environmental toxicology, in both of these situations the dose (*D*) is replaced by concentration (*C*). These indices are expressed as EC_x or LC_x values with the duration of exposure additionally included in the definition.

For completeness, and to avoid confusion, it must be noted that that the LD_x and LC_x nomenclature are occasionally used in sub-acute and long-term toxicology but when this happens the circumstances generally preclude ambiguity[171].

In a typical sub-acute investigation involving lethality, animals are exposed daily (i.e. either daily dosing or continuously in the diet or atmosphere) for a set period of time; mortality is recorded on a daily basis for each exposure (*note*: in experiments involving daily dosing it is important to record whether death occurred before or after that day's exposure). With daily dosing experiments it is important that the animals are exposed at the same time each day. Table 3.2 is a simple, hypothetical, example in which a chemical is administered daily (at 24 hourly intervals) to groups of 10 animals.

Table 3.2 Hypothetical data illustrating a typical pattern for mortality occurring during a sub-acute toxicity investigation

Dose $mg\ kg^{-1}\ day^{-1}$	Mortality (group size = 10)			
	Day 1	Day 2	Day 3	Day 4 . . . etc
5	0	0	0	1
10	0	0	1	5
20	0	2	6	9
40	0	4	8	10

It could be concluded that the single dose LD_{50} value for this chemical was greater than 40 mg kg^{-1} but that it exhibits some degree of cumulative toxicity so that with 4 consecutive days exposure the 'sub-acute LD_{50} value' was approximately 10 mg kg^{-1} day^{-1} and so on. These quantitative changes in LD_{50} values with exposures taking place over a period of time are sometimes used as indices of cumulative toxicity[171,393,683] and the derivation of these, so called, 'chronicity index' values is described later in this chapter.

The underlying principles of quantification in acute toxicology owe much to the ideas of biological assays for pharmacologically active drugs that could not be assayed chemically. Usually the work of Trevan[172] is cited as the first definitive publication in this field but arguably there were earlier relevant papers[173] that could have led to the same general conclusions. The difficulties associated with using the minimum lethal dose (i.e. the threshold dose) were recognized by Trevan[172]. Three major and many lesser variables are associated with the toxicity of any product. The major variables are:

(a) The nature and amount of the toxicant
The toxicokinetics and the toxicodynamics of any product are intimately related to its physical–chemical characteristics and the form in which it is presented to the target. The quantity of toxicant involved is generally called the 'dose' or the 'exposure level'. To define dose, or exposure level, the most usual units are the weights, or occasionally volumes of the toxicants. There are occasions when it is expedient to express the exposure as moles of toxicants rather than by weight or volume (*note*: moles are generally used when comparisons are being made between different congeners in QSAR studies and also to express the acute toxicities of molecules that may be presented to targets in different chemical forms, such as different salts).

For dynamic exposures (e.g. inhalation toxicology, aquatic toxicology, etc.) the amounts of toxicants are generally expressed in terms of environmental concentrations.

It is sometimes desirable to estimate the actual amount of a gaseous toxicant taken in by an animal and this requires the application of both physico–chemical as well as physiological principles[635]. A general formula for the estimation of retained dose in inhalation exposure situations is:

$$\text{retained dose} \quad = \quad \frac{CtV_m\alpha}{W} \text{ mg kg}^{-1}$$

where C = concentration of toxicant (mg m^{-3})
  t = duration of exposure (min.)
  V_m = minute volume for animal (m^3 min^{-1})
  α = retention coefficient (decimal notation)
  W = body weight (kg)

but, if concentration of gas in the atmosphere is expressed in parts per million (ppm), then to obtain C the following calculation must be used:

$$C = \frac{\text{conc.(ppm)} \times \text{mol. mass of gas}}{\text{Avogadro's Constant*}} \text{ mg m}^{-3}$$

(b) Duration of exposure

For the majority of acute situations the toxicant enters the target organism as a one-off amount, sometimes called a 'bolus', and the duration of exposure can be considered to be infinitely short. Duration of exposure must not be confused with the duration of residence of the toxicant molecule within target organism or with the duration of the response. Both duration of residence and duration of response are extremely important and influence acute toxicology in relation to antidotal treatment[174-176].

There are some exposures in acute toxicology that are not of the one-off amount (bolus) type. Some exceptions are:

(i)   repeated exposures within time span of 24 hours,
(ii) depot dosage,
(iii) slow infusion dosage and
(iv) continuous dynamic exposure

Definitions of exposures associated with slow infusion or with continuous dynamic situations necessitate specification of the duration of exposure. For repeated exposures within 24 hours the sub-division of the amounts and time intervals should be specified as this may affect the findings. Depot dosage is mostly limited to certain types of medicaments (e.g. drug implants) or to materials used for prostheses and, for the purpose of acute toxicology, the duration of exposure cannot be effectively defined.

Sub-acute exposures may be continuous over a period of time or, more often, a sequence of individual exposures. In the latter case the interval time between each exposure may be of paramount importance to the toxic sequalae as the response may be dependent on the quantity of toxicant or its metabolites remaining in the animal from the previous exposure or exposures; the rate of metabolism and excretion of the toxicant are clearly critical factors. From this statement it is immediately apparent that any predictive sub-acute toxicology experiment involving the use of repeated exposures in animals must be designed with the intervals between exposures standardized, (*note*: the choice of time interval will not necessarily be the same for all investigations and must be considered carefully by the investigator) or the findings may be confounded.

---

*This is 22.4 at standard temperature and pressure (STP); this figure has to be adjusted for the ambient conditions of the exposure.

Perhaps less apparent than the obvious selection of exposure times in individual dosing regimens is the fact that exposure in food or drinking water is not continuous exposure, animals do not eat or drink all of the time, nor even at regular intervals, therefore intake of toxicant is not well controlled by the investigator.

(c) Characteristics of the exposed organism

It is expedient in acute and sub-acute toxicology to relate exposures to the body weights of the animals involved. Exposure, or dose, is most often expressed in terms of the quantity (generally the weight) of toxicant per unit body weight of the exposed animals. The amount of toxicant is commonly expressed in milligrams and the unit of body weight as one kilogram. Occasionally units other than milligrams for the toxicant and one kilogramme for the body weight are used, and it is imperative that these units are clearly specified.

It is usual for the dose or exposure to be written in the form:

$mg\ kg^{-1}$ or mg/kg

and if time is included, these are expanded to:

$mg\ kg^{-1}\ day^{-1}$ or mg/kg/day

using the appropriate time unit (i.e. seconds, minutes, hours, etc.) and stating the total duration. Thus it might be stated that 'chemical A was administered at the rate of 25 $mg\ kg^{-1}\ day^{-1}$ (or 25 mg/kg/day) for 14 consecutive days'.

Sometimes in sub-acute toxicology exposures are to diets containing the toxicant. The amounts of toxicant in the diet are generally expressed as 'parts per million (ppm)'. It is fairly common practice for investigators to calculate an amount of toxicant consumed per day from the weighed food intake of the animals. It must be realized that the resulting figures are imprecise but, provided that the experiments have been done with adequate attention to detail (e.g. allowance made for food lost due to scattering rather than actually being consumed), then the results are generally within acceptable limits. The calculation of intakes of toxicants from gaseous atmospheres, also measured in ppm, are more complex and are dealt with on page 38.

Allometric principles suggest reasonably simple relationships between the dimensions of body surface and body weight[177,178] but some caution is necessary in the acceptance of these relationships as being absolutely correct[179-185,648,650]. Correlations between physiological functions and body weight or body surface area are more complex and less absolute than might appear to be the case[186,649,650]. None the less ideas of correlations between exposure, body weight and response meet acceptable criteria in practice[187,649].

There are essentially two reasons for considering that body surface area is important in acute toxicology; firstly there are some chemicals for which it is found that there are better functional correlations between exposure, body surface area and response than exist between exposure, body weight and response[188-190,650]. The second reason relates to the caution that must be applied to allometric interrelationships associated with the transition from juvenile to adult in any vertebrate species[191,648,686].

There are some products that do not appear to exert their toxic effects in a way that is dose-related to either body weight or to body surface area. Two published examples of chemicals that appear to exert their toxicities in ways that are not related to either body weight or surface area are the rodenticide alphanaphthylthiourea (ANTU) in the wild Norway rat[192,193] and in some species, the toxin associated with *Clostridium botulinum*[195,196]. In predictive acute toxicity testing it is necessary to be cautious about the apparent lack of relationship between exposure, body weight (or body surface area) and response as this can sometimes be an artefact associated with the experimental design (e.g. size of the experimental population)[194]. With this, and as a general principle, investigators must always be suspicious of findings that do not conform to expected biological patterns; confirmation of exceptions is a prerequisite of investigative toxicology.

It is very difficult to determine threshold exposure levels in acute toxicology but clearly there must be such a value for each toxicant in every individual animal. This truism can be expressed symbolically as follows; if Th is the threshold level for the toxic response to just occur and Z is the dose, or exposure level:

then, if $Z \geq Th$ response will occur
and if $Z < Th$ response will not occur.

The threshold value (Th) is associated with a composite of metabolic characteristics and not with body weight or body surface area alone[197]. Although it might seem to be an attractive concept, no universally acceptable 'metabolic body weight' has yet been devised[181,648]. It is known that the threshold level (Th) is a random variable throughout any exposed population. This randomness is the fundamental property that allows quantification of acute toxicity in the form of indices such as LD_{50} values.

The idea of effect dose (ED) and lethal dose (LD) as quantitative entities is not peculiar to the assessment of acute toxicity in vertebrates but has close comparability to measurements used by microbiologists. Because of the nature of their test organisms microbiologists are able to carry out investigations with very large populations and this has obvious statistical advantages over the much smaller populations available to investigators in acute toxicology.

Following on from the publication in 1927 by Trevan[172] it is usually accepted that the next major contribution relevant to the biometrics of acute toxicology was a publication by Bliss in 1935[198]. Some of the key points from this outstanding publication are:

(a) The dose–mortality relationship is primarily descriptive of the variation in susceptibility between individuals within the population.
(b) Susceptibility varies from one individual to another.
(c) The distribution curve of the number of individuals having each particular susceptibility will have the shape characteristics of the normal curve of error (note: a bell-shaped curve as shown in Figure 3.1).

Since it is not possible to determine the threshold dose (Th) for each individual animal, the idea of studying the effect of the product quantitatively in groups of animals becomes important (i.e. population effects). Groups of animals can be exposed to specified dose levels of the product and the number of individuals within each group either exhibiting or not exhibiting the defined response can be counted. If several groups of animals, exposed at different dose levels, are used it is possible to deduce a relationship between exposure and response. For the majority of products it can be accepted that the relationship between exposure and response (expressed as a proportion of the population responding) takes the

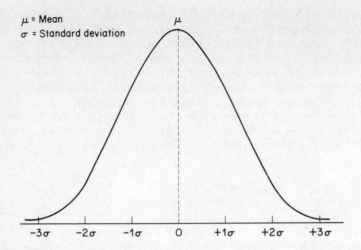

Fig. 3.1   A typical distribution curve of the number of individuals in a population exhibiting a particular susceptibility.

form of a sigmoid curve when both variables are plotted as linear graphs, (a typical example is illustrated in Figure 3.2)[199]. The numbers of animals used in the majority of acute toxicity tests are insufficient to establish the sigmoid relationship but it is assumed, *a priori*, that the data would fulfill this criterion[615].

Many biologists find that biometric sigmoid curves are difficult to interpret and this difficulty is accentuated when the available data is insufficient to permit the sigmoid curve to be plotted with certainty[617]. The ideas of data transformation from one scale to another is not novel and in the nineteenth century it was recognized that biological variation often fits logarithmic rather than arithmetic characteristics[200,201]. The effect of transforming dose–response data to log–linear form is not simply to modify, but retain, the sigmoid shape and this is not helpful with interpretation of the data.

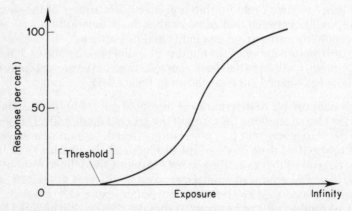

Fig. 3.2   A typical sigmoid curve obtained when both exposure and response are plotted on linear coordinates.

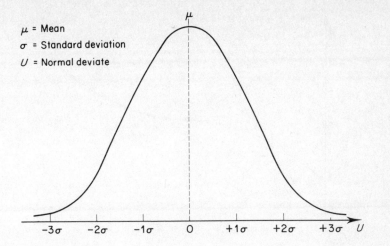

μ = Mean
σ = Standard deviation
U = Normal deviate

Fig. 3.3 A typical distribution curve showing the normal deviate (U) from which the normal equivalent deviate may be derived.

The problem of relating response to dose in simplified form was of interest to pharmacologists and biometricians concerned with the development of bioassays for products that could not be assayed by chemical analysis (e.g. cardio-active components of digitalis extracts, some hormones, etc). Researching bioassay procedures, Gaddum[202] described a statistical variate which he called the 'normal equivalent deviate' (*NED*). The *NED* is derived from the normal distribution curve (Figure 3.3) and it is the value on the abscissa which marks off proportions p and $(1 - p)$ of the normal distribution. Since the midpoint of the normal curve must correspond to an abscissa value of zero, then values of p that are less than one-half correspond to negative *NED*'s and values of p that are greater than one-half correspond to positive *NED*'s. The *NED* (Figure 3.3) can be expressed as:

$$NED = \frac{1}{\sqrt{2\pi}} \int_{-\infty}^{y} \exp\left(-\tfrac{1}{2}U^2\right) dU$$

Gaddum[202] further devised a means by which the use of the *NED* could be simplified by abolishing negative values. Gaddum's new unit, was called the 'probit' (the word 'probit' is derived from the abbreviated combination of two words, 'probability' and 'unit') and is quite simply obtained by the addition of five to each *NED* value:

any probit value = (corresponding *NED* value + 5)

or in mathematical terms:

$$NED = \frac{1}{\sqrt{2\pi}} \int_{-\infty}^{(y-5)} \exp\left(-\tfrac{1}{2}U^2\right) dU$$

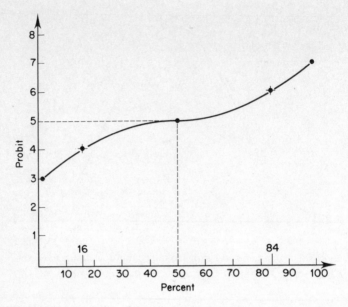

Fig. 3.4   A graphical presentation of the relationship between percentage values and probits.

The symmetrical relationship between probit values and their corresponding percentage values can be seen if they are plotted as a graph (Figure 3.4). Tabulations of percentages with corresponding probit values are included in many books of statistical tables and Finney[203] has published the definitive account of the derivation of probit analysis and its applications in biometrics. If, instead of simple log–linear transform of the dose without transformation of response, the same data are subjected to double transformation, in other words, doses plotted on log scale and responses plotted as probits, then the data shown in Figure 3.2 assumes an approximately straight line form (Figure 3.5). There is minimum deviation from this straight line relationships at the mid-point (i.e. the point corresponding to probit value 5, the 50% population response) and the magnitude of the deviation increases towards the extreme points (i.e. towards the points corresponding to zero and 100% response levels).

Two pairs of investigators must be credited with the firm establishment of the graphical approach to the handling of acute toxicity data by the use of probit analysis. Miller and Tainter[204] proposed a simple graphical approach and a few years later their technique was expanded by Litchfield and Wilcoxon[205]. The techniques attributed to these investigators are still widely used, and are critically acknowledged by many toxicologists[615,622].

Probit analysis may be performed graphically but programmable electronic calculators and computers have made it convenient to calculate acute toxicity data without the need for graphs. The underlying principles are the same and it is easy to build useful refinements into the program. Several programs for probit analysis have been published[206-209]. If the graphical approach is used the data may be plotted by the line of best fit[211], as seen by eye, but it is more bio-

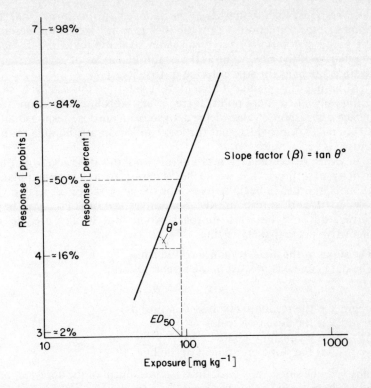

Fig. 3.5 A typical dose–response line for an acute toxicity investigation (response plotted on Probit scale and exposure plotted on log-scale).

metrically acceptable to apply regression techniques to the whole data from all of the dose response groups[210,617]. Because of the non-linear, albeit symmetrical, transformation of the response data to probit values it is not valid to apply simple linear regression methods in probit analysis but other suitable regression techniques are available and should be included in any program for non-graphical calculation of acute toxicity data[206-209].

The most important interpretative aspects of acute data, when handled by probit analysis, are as follows:

(a) The effect doses

Provided that extreme point data are excluded (i.e. those data corresponding to nil response and 100% response) then a minimum of three data points are required to fit a line to a graph of the type shown in Figure 3.5 or to carry out the comparable calculation using a suitable program. Simple numeric principles make it clear that more than three data points would enable a better judgement of the line of best fit but that a minimum of three data points is workable provided that the points are well spaced out on the scale[211]. Also, it is essential that the response points are distributed on both sides of the mid-point (i.e. both sides of the probit value 5 or 50% response level). The confidence that can be attributed to any points on the dose–response line diminishes as the data gets further away from the mid-point in either direction[212], thus the 50% response is the most defensible of the numeric criteria for use as an index of acute toxicity[213,214], hence the popularity of the LD_{50} value as the established index of acute toxicity when death is taken as the sole criterion of toxicity.

Although the median lethal dose level (i.e. the LD_{50}) is the most commonly used data-point there is no absolute objection to other percentage response values being derived from the dose-response data, (e.g. LD_{10} or LD_{80}), provided that the lesser precision attributable to the value chosen is acceptable[213,214].

In order to establish a meaningful threshold dose level for the acute toxicity of a product it would be necessary to use huge populations of animals in order to begin to overcome the error factor associated with the low end of the dose response line. Some investigations of this type have been carried out[215-218] but this approach would not be favoured in normal predictive acute toxicity testing.

(b) The slope of the dose–response relationship

The data can be expressed in the algebraic form:

$$y = a + bx$$

where y is the response (expressed in probits)

   x is the dose (log scale)

   a is a constant (characteristic of the line)

   b is the slope or gradient of the line

thus, b, the slope, may be defined by the tangent of the dose–response line in relation to the abscissa

because the doubly transformed dose–response relationship approximates to a straight line.

The numeric value of the gradient (b) is used as an index of the slope characteristic of the dose–response line. It is common practice to refer to 'steep' or to 'shallow' dose–response, depending on whether the value of 'b' is large or small. Examples of steep dose–response relationships were found by Klonne and co-workers[640] during their investigations of the acute inhalation toxicology of a series of aliphatic nitrites; these investigators concluded that these volatile nitrites are commonly found among glues and solvents[652,653] inhaled by some people to create a 'high' (i.e. a form of addictive abuse). The actual median lethal doses (LC_{50} values) might create a false sense of safety for these nitrites are considerably more hazardous, because of their dose–response characteristics, than is apparent from their LC_{50} values.

The insecticide endrin has been investigated as a toxicant in many different species and has been found, in some, to exhibit a shallow dose–response relationship[687].

Because the choice of exposure levels for use in sub-acute investigations can only be based on available information and such information is often restricted to data from acute tests, it is essential for the investigators to take into account the slope characteristics of the acute response. It is common practice for sub-acute exposure levels to be chosen on the basis of defined fractions of the LD_{50} value; obviously the intrinsic meanings of fractions of LD_{50} values will be greatly affected by the slope characteristics.

The characteristics of the dose–response line have important applications in acute toxicology:

(i)   *Safety*. Any number of products may have the same LD_{50} value but their slope characteristics may be quite different. If the slope is 'steep' then a small diminution in the exposure level will still have the effect of substantially reducing the number of animals that will be killed but if the slope is 'shallow' it will necessitate a much smaller exposure to substantially reduce the number of animals killed. In other words, even if different products have the same LD_{50} value they may possess very different thresholds of acute toxicity and this lethal potential may be critically important in relation to safety.

(ii) *Interactive Effects*. Multiple exposure to different, or even the same chemicals can influence responses. The different types of interactive effect are discussed in Section 3.3.

(iii) *Confidence Limits*. Since all quantitative estimates of acute toxicity are based on dose–response relationships in populations, they are at best, only statistically derived estimates based on probability. Because of the derivation of the data it is statistically acceptable to assume that the error associated with any point on the dose–response line will be symmetrically distributed about the mean value for the particular point; graphically the error distribution takes the bell-shaped curve form (Figure 3.1) and 95% of the area under such curves is contained within an area bounded by $\pm$ 1.96 standard deviations. In toxicology it is an accepted convention that confidence limits are nearly always calculated at the 95% probability level (*note*: this is often presented in the alternative form, $P = 0.95$).

To achieve 95% confidence limits for any point on the dose–response line it is necessary to calculate the standard error for the particular point and then to multiply this value by 1.96, (i.e. the number of standard deviations that bound 95% of the values):

If μ =   mean value of dose–response

σ =   standard deviation

n =   number of animals

then,

$$\frac{\sigma}{\sqrt{n}} = \text{standard error of mean}$$

hence, the mean with 95% confidence limits is,

$$\mu \pm \frac{1.96\sigma}{\sqrt{n}}$$

Translating this information into words; 'The best estimate of the mean value from the available dose–response data is μ and, statistically, if the test were to be repeated in identical form it may be anticipated that the mean estimate would lie between $\mu \pm \dfrac{(1.96)\sigma}{\sqrt{n}}$ for 95 out of 100 times that the test is conducted.'

To illustrate this statement by means of an example the following is taken from a publication[219] on the acute toxicology of tropilidene: 'The single dose acute oral LD_{50} value of undiluted tropilidene was found to be 171 mg kg^{-1} (95% confidence limits, 153 to 190 mg kg^{-1}) in CFNol strain mice.' This statement means that under the specified conditions the best estimate for the single dose acute oral LD_{50} value for tropilidene in mice of the CFNol strain was 171 mg kg^{-1}. Statistically it can be assumed that if the test is replicated, under exactly the same conditions, then for 95 out of every 100 replicates the mean value of the LD_{50} would be expected to fall between 153 and 190 mg kg^{-1} or, conversely, 5 times in each 100 replicates the mean may be outside those limits.

It is most important not to attribute any additional meaning to confidence limits outside their relationship to the data from the specific investigation. Confidence limits do not give any indication of the intrinsic quality of the data obtained during the investigation and they apply only to exact replicates of the experimental conditions.

The calculations of confidence limits and slope factors are easily achieved by means of programs for calculators or computers[672]. Examination of one graphical method[205], without mathematical proof, illustrates the ease with which these calculations can be performed:

First determine the doses corresponding to the responses for probit values 4 and 6 (i.e. these are equivalent to values of LD_{16} and LD_{84}),
Then calculate the slope function (S) when;

$$S = \left[\frac{LD_{84}}{LD_{50}} + \frac{LD_{50}}{LD_{16}} \right] \times \frac{1}{2}$$

If N is the number of animals used in the investigation for the exposure levels between (and including) the LD_{16} and the LD_{84}, then;

$$S^{\text{exponent}} = S^{\frac{2.77}{\sqrt{N}}} = \text{Function of } LD_{50}$$

and the confidence limits at the 95% probability level are given by:

[lower limit] $\dfrac{LD_{50}}{\text{function of } LD_{50}}$ [upper limit] $LD_{50} \times \text{function of } LD_{50}$

A simple method that does not require the same number of animals to be used for each exposure level, but does require the successive dose intervals to be geometrically constant, was devised by Karber[220]. Unlike probit analysis it is a requirement of Karber's method that the exposure range for the test must include both extreme points (i.e. nil and 100% response). The formula for calculating the LD_{50} value (ED_{50} value) can be written as:

$$\text{Log } LD_{50} = \text{Log } LD_{100} - \left[\frac{R_1 + R_2}{2} + \frac{R_2 + R_3}{2} + \frac{R_3 + R_4}{2} + \ldots \right] \times d$$

when, LD_{100} is defined as the smallest dose in the investigations that kills all animals, $R_1, R_2, R_3 \ldots$ are the responses expressed in decimal notation (i.e. on the scale of 0 to 1 for nil response to 100% response). 'd' is the dose interval which is the ratio between successive exposure levels.

Having done this simple calculation the LD_{50} value is the anti-logarithm of the calculated answer. This method provides a convenient approximation only. The method has been criticized by biometricians[222,223,615] and it has been modified[224] but, even so, it is useful if used with an awareness of its limitations. Serious limitations to the investigator are the inability of Karber's method to reveal information on the slope factor and also its failure to provide confidence limits[615].

Probit analysis has provided the most widely used approach to the calculation of data from acute toxicity testing but there are other, less frequently used transformations that can be applied to these data. Angular transformation[225] and logistic functions[226] have both been used and Rybach and co-workers[227] developed ideas based on stochastic approximations and the stochastic approach has been endorsed by other biometricians as a means for handling quantal data in toxicology[167].

The most widely used alternative to probit analysis for acute toxicity data is generally called the method of 'moving averages'. The concept of 'moving averages' was published by W. R. Thompson in 1947 and was later reviewed in a publication by Armitage and Allen[223]. Subsequent to these publications more detailed tables for use with the method were made available in the literature[212,228,229]. The method of moving averages establishes a reasonable estimate of LD_{50} values provided that two essential requirements are met: firstly, there must be the same number of animals in each exposure group and secondly, the interval between successive exposure levels must be geometrically constant. Given that these two criteria are fulfilled then:

$$m = \log D + \frac{d(k+1)}{2} + dF$$

m = logarithm of the median effect dose (M)
if D = lowest exposure level tested
d = logarithm of ratio of successive doses
F = value obtained from tables[212,228,229]
$(K + 1)$ = total number of exposure levels tested
and M = antilog m.

The confidence limits (95% probability level) are then calculated in terms of the logarithmic values;
$m \pm$ factor d
the factor 'd' is obtainable from computed tables[212,228,229]
thus LD_{50} value = antilog $m = M$
and the confidence limits (95% probability level) are given by:
antilog ($m \pm$ factor d).
Good agreement between LD_{50} values calculated by the method of moving averages and other methods has been established[230]. It has also been demonstrated that it is possible to obtain realistic slope factors using the moving averages method with only a few animals in each exposure group[221,230].

The '**Up and Down**' method (alternatively called the '**Pyramid**' method) for determining LD_{50} values has been around for quite a long time[655] but its popularity with toxicologists has tended to be limited to investigations involving the use of large or expensive animals[574]. The 'Up and Down' method starts with two levels of exposure, one being high and the other low, with very small numbers of animals in each group (n.b. on occasions some investigators have found one animal at each level to be sufficient for their needs). After the required time for observation has elapsed, and this will vary with the nature of the toxicant, further exposure levels are started sequentially, either higher or lower, until the median lethal dose is reached[655-659].

The principal merit of the 'Up and Down' approach to testing is the small number of animals used when compared with the much larger numbers required for conventional LD_{50} tests. Some investigators, comparing data on the same toxicants tested conventionally and by the 'Up and Down' method, have reported excellent agreement between the findings and that the number of animals needed was only 6 to 9 for a product in the 'Up and Down' method but was 40 to 50 in the formal LD_{50} test procedure[660,661]. The disadvantages of the 'Up and Down' approach are that it is slow to complete because it is sequential and that the final results are not statistically elegant; current thinking suggests that this latter point may not be a serious disadvantage[569-575].

Within the context of quantification there has been some recognition of the idea that acute toxicity may be more complex than an 'all or none' response hence the polychotomous quantal response takes cognizance of more complicated sequences, such as alive-moribund-dead (a trichotomous sequence), when there is a defined order of outcomes. The easiest method for handling polychotomous data depends on its reduction to dichomotous form by the sequential pooling of data. For the trichotomous form which is the polychotomous response most frequently met in acute toxicology:

alive → moribund → dead

becomes,   alive → (moribund and dead)

and asymptotically efficient estimators, such as maximum likelihood or minimum chi-Square techniques, can be applied to the data[231-233].

Sometimes in experimental acute toxicity testing it is found that data does not fit an expected dose–response pattern[192-194]. This lack of conformity is often attributable to experimental flaws but, sometimes, the lack of obvious dose–response relationship may be due to polymorphic relationships[234-236]. If the dose–response is truly polymorphic then it is not correct to estimate an LD_{50} value, but the alternative possibility involving aberrant experimental results must be thoroughly investigated before any final conclusions are established.

Quantification in sub-acute toxicology may take the form of detailed investigations of changes that occur in such things as body weight, organ weights, physiological chemistry variables, haematological values, etc. If the investigation is to include considerations of these changes then it is imperative that the experimental protocol is designed to include the statistical analyses that will inevitably follow. If the investigation is not designed with adequate attention to size of treatment groups, statistical randomization of animals within and between groups, etc, then the findings may be erroneous and misleading. Some sub-acute studies in predictive toxicology are less detailed and may be adequate; the investigator must consider the needs at the outset, these may be influenced by the class of product being investigated.

A major use of sub-acute toxicity tests is to assess cumulative toxicity potential. There is a school of thought that the best way of quantifying cumulative toxicity potential is to create an index value based on the sub-acute toxicity rating determined as a cumulative LD_{50} value and the single dose, acute, LD_{50} value. Boyd[393] proposed a cumulative toxicity index based on the repeated dose sub-acute LD_{50} value with the number of repeat doses, at daily intervals, being over a period equivalent to one-tenth of the expected life span for the test species, (*note*: One-tenth of the life span is the accepted convention for the maximum duration of a sub-acute toxicity test). If, in shortened form, this is written as:

[0.1*l*] LD_{50} value where *l* is the life span in years
and the single dose LD_{50} value, by the same route, in comparable animals:
[SD] LD_{50} value
then, Boyd's Chronicity Index was expressed as:

$$\frac{[0.1l] \ LD_{50} \text{ value in mg kg}^{-1} \text{ day}^{-1}}{[SD] \ LD_{50} \text{ value in mg kg}^{-1}} = \text{Chronicity Index [Boyd]}$$

A modification of Boyd's approach was proposed by Hayes[683] and this was essentially a reciprocal of Boyd's index. Some would argue that chronicity indices of these types have limited meaning. The main objections can be summarized as follows:

(a) LD_{50} values carry wide confidence limits thus basing everything on ratios of the calculated median doses may be misleading.
(b) Chronicity indices only measure cumulative effect and not cumulative storage.
(c) The only cumulative effect that is measured is death. The cumulative toxicology of a product might include important sub-lethal effects.
(d) The single dose LD_{50} values are generally obtained in animals following a period without food whereas the sub-acute LD_{50} value cannot be obtained in this way. Thus comparisons between the two sets of data are artificial.

At best chronicity indices, of the type described, should be considered as being a crude guide to the occurrence of cumulative toxicity. Too much importance should not be attached to the actual numeric values obtained.

3.3 Interactive effects

To facilitate understanding of toxicology it is expedient to consider interactions of one moiety with the target species in isolation from all other chemical interference whereas, in reality, the target species is never exposed to only one chemical in isolation[237]. Even if nothing else all animals are exposed to food and other environmental chemicals and the possibility that seemingly innocuous products might influence the toxicology of other chemicals cannot be disregarded[684]. Ingestion of foods containing tyramine by people being treated with monoamine oxidase inhibitors as anti-depressants and the toxic sequalae is one well documented example of this aspect of acute toxicology[238]; there are many others[684].

In terms of serious acute intoxication many multiple exposures do not exhibit overt interactions but this does not rule out the possibility of subtle effects occurring. However, some multiple exposures profoundly affect the outcome of intoxication; it is convenient to consider interactions as being of four main types although overlaps between the types are common occurrences:

(i) Chemical interactions

Some toxicant molecules behave quite differently if they have interacted with other chemical moieties although the original toxicant molecule may still be essentially intact. This phenomenon is commonly observed with toxicants that are bases; reaction of bases with acids, to form salts, may completely change the toxicokinetic characteristics of the parent base molecule. This same principle applies to many other interactions and this is sometimes used quite deliberately to change the pharmacokinetic characteristics of therapeutic agents or the applicability of pesticides, thus improving efficacy as well as influencing toxicity.

(ii) Physiological effects

Interference with the physiology of the target organism by one or more chemicals may influence the acute toxicity potential of another product.

Skin penetration by a toxicant may be enhanced or retarded by the action of chemicals on the skin. For example, the percutaneous acute toxicity of many pesticides is enhanced by formulation in various solvents and these affect the skin by degreasing or causing epidermal damage and sometimes by increasing blood flow in the cutaneous vascular bed[239]. Skin is not the only organ that can be physiologically altered to influence acute toxicity for the alimentary tract is also susceptible to alteration. The timing of food intake in relation to ingestion of a toxicant can markedly affect absorption and for some products the effect will be a slowing of uptake and with others the rate of uptake may be increased[240,619]. Co-administration of a large volume of fluid often facilitates uptake of toxicants from the digestive tract but this will be influenced by the nature of the fluid[241].

In predictive acute toxicity testing it is common practice to withhold food from test animals for a period of several hours prior to administration of the test material[620]; if the test product cannot be administered undiluted it is given either as a solution or suspension, in what may be a large volume of liquid relative to the normal alimentary intake. The findings from predictive tests must always take into account withholding food and also the influence of fluid intake on the toxicology of the product being tested[154,241,242,619,620].

Excretion of toxicants and metabolites can also be influenced by interactive physiological effects. Pharmacological acidification of the urine decreases the excretion of weakly acidic toxicants (e.g. phenobarbitone) but increases the excretion of basic toxicants (e.g. many alkaloids); conversely changing the urinary pH to alkaline has the opposite effects. Quite apart from urinary pH effects some chemicals are capable of affecting the active transport systems in the kidneys and these products may cause retention or alternatively more rapid elimination of the toxicant; the uricosuric drug probenecid is an example of a compound that can markedly affect the excretion of other toxicants or drugs[238].

(iii) Biochemical effects

There are many chemicals that cause induction of the hepatic enzymes and the overall influence of enzyme induction is to change the rate of metabolism of any xenobiotic that is toxified, or detoxified, by the particular enzyme systems that have been induced. Enzyme inducers are ubiquitous so that some degree of enzyme induction occurs in all animals. In investigative toxicology it is essential to avoid adventitiously exposing animals to potent inducers. For example, dieldrin, a potent inducer of hepatic enzymes, has been widely used for the preservative treatment of wood and it is quite possible for some animals to be in close contact with dieldrin treated wood products as part of their normal husbandry[243,244]. Many humans are likely to be exposed to potent enzyme inducers, (e.g. phenobarbitone a widely used drug), and these can influence sensitivity to toxicants.

Enzyme inducers can exert an auto-toxic effect. For example, previous exposure of an animal to barbiturates may diminish sensitivity to further barbiturate exposure thus increasing the amount of the barbiturate required to cause acute intoxication[238].

Toxification, or detoxification, mechanisms are largely dependent on the multiplicity of enzymes that are present in the exposed animal. Some toxicants exert their action by inhibiting one or more of the enzyme systems (e.g. inhibition of various cholinesterases by some organophosphorus compounds) and sometimes this inhibition of enzymes by toxicant influences sensitivity to subsequent intoxication by other products. This effect is apparent if disulfiram is administered to humans; the disulfiram inhibits aldehyde dehydrogenase but appears to have little toxic effect unless there is subsequent exposure to ethanol. The acute manifestations of ethanol exposure after disulfiram are very apparent and are due to the systemic build-up of acetaldehyde:

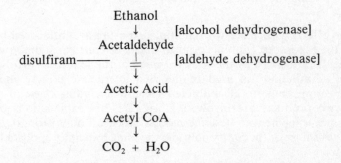

The symptomatology of ethanol intoxication in subjects pre-treated with disulfiram include; increased heart rate, sweating, breathlessness, headache, vomitting, dizziness, an initial rise in blood pressure followed by hypertension sometimes leading to fatal shock. Disulfiram provides an interesting example of the importance of adventitious interactions in acute toxicology for, apart from its use as a therapeutic agent, disulfiram has been used in the rubber processing industries and the symptomatology described has occurred among occupationally exposed process workers.

Organophosphorus and carbamate compounds are both widely used as insecticides. This use is dependent on the ability of these chemicals to inhibit cholinesterase enzymes in insects. This same enzyme inhibitory property is primarily responsible for their toxicity in vertebrate animals and it is often found that previous exposure to one of these agents increases sensitivity to intoxication by subsequent exposure to another anticholinesterase agent[245-247]. This increased sensitivity to intoxication is potentially dangerous for people, and other animals, who may be repeatedly exposed to pesticides because of agricultural practices or for those concerned with manufacturing, formulating, transporting and packaging agricultural chemicals, thus stringent precautions must be used to avoid interactive intoxication by these products.

Occasionally biphasic effects of chemicals on enzyme systems occur. When this happens the enzyme inhibitory effects of exposure to a chemical are supplemented by enzyme induction. If the exposure continues for long enough it may have an effect on the potential acute toxicity of any other chemicals to which the animal may be exposed. This biphasic phenomenon is sometimes observed in the acute toxicology of organophosphorus anti-cholinesterase agents, the primary toxic effect being inhibition of cholines-terases and the secondary toxic effect resulting from enzyme inductions[248-250]. The importance of this interactive relationship, together with an analysis of the various mechanisms involved, have been reviewed by Cohen[251] and it is apparent that interactive effects may be occurring at levels of exposure below those needed to cause overt signs of cholinergic response.

(iv) Physical effects

The acute toxic potential of any product may be substantially influenced by the physical conditions associated with the exposure. Some of the effects of ambient conditions are discussed in Section 3.4 but here physical effects may be exemplified by the influence of occlusive covering on percutaneous absorption[93] and the influence of partial pressure on the uptake of gaseous toxicants[252].

Interactive effects associated with multiple exposure are influenced by the sequence of the exposures. Multiple exposures may be concurrent or sequential and the effect is influenced by the relative timing of the sequences involved.

A specific terminology is used to describe interactive effects and this terminology is applicable to all multiple exposures including those in which more than two products are involved[677]. To facilitate explanations of the terminology it is expedient to describe models based on only two interacting products but this is done for clarity only and the same principles apply to larger numbers:

Consider two products A and B: The responses to acute exposure to each of two products are expressed as 'effects of A' and 'effects of B' respectively. Exposure to both of the products A and B can give rise to any of the following five possibilities;

(a) Additive Effect. This is the simplest situation in which there is no apparent interaction at all. The responses to A and B are independent of each other and this model can be written as:

'effect of A' + 'effect of B' = 'effect of (A + B)'

(b) Synergistic Effect (Synergism). Literally synergism means 'working with cooperation'. If any two products A and B have similar modes of action and the resulting effect from exposure, whether concurrent or consecutive, to both A and B is greater than would be expected from the sum of the individual effects, then this increased response is termed synergism. This may be written as:

'effect of (A + B)' > 'effect of A' + 'effect of B'

(c) **Potentiation**. Potentiation is said to occur if A and B have different modes of action and the effect due to exposure, either concurrently or consecutively, to the two products is greater than would be expected for the individual components A or B. The model, as presented below, appears to be identical to that for a synergistic effect,

'effect of (A + B)' > 'effect of A' + 'effect of B'

but the essential difference lies in the relationship of the modes of action of the individual products A and B.

It is a fine point of definition as to what is really meant by 'similar' or 'different' modes of action (*note*: the definition may be confounded by the fact that many products exhibit more than one mode of toxic action and these may be influenced by the exposure level) and it is not uncommon to find the terms 'synergism' and 'potentiation' being used as if they are synonymous. This confusion of terminology is often displayed in the labelling of domestic aerosol packs of insecticides where synthetic or natural derivatives of pyrethrum are said to be 'synergised' with piperonyl butoxide, or similar agents; both in relation to toxicity to insects and to vertebrates the modes of action of the pyrethroid components and the piperonyl butoxide are dissimilar and therefore the enhancing effect is really potentiation and not synergism.

(d) **Coalitive Effects.** Theoretically it is possible for the toxic response resulting from concurrent exposure to the two products A and B to be different from the responses due to either A or B alone. This situation occurs so rarely that it is of little more than theoretical interest[253,254]. The model for coalitive effects may be written as

'effect of (A + B)' independent of 'effect of A' + 'effect of B.'

Investigators are advised that if a coalitive effect is thought to have occurred in relation to the toxicology of a multiple exposure then the modes of action of each of the components should be carefully reappraised before any final conclusion is reached. A likely explanation of this rare event would be the unveiling of biphasic responses by the individual components.

(e) **Antagonism.** Antagonism is a general term that describes the situation when the response to A and B is less than the effects of either component. That is

'effect of (A + B)' < 'effect of A' + 'effect of B'.

The term antagonism may be used whatever the mode of action of A and B on each other provided that the overall response is less than additive.

In toxicology antagonism may occur in numerous different ways. For example, one component of the interaction may block toxicant–receptor interaction in the target (e.g. chlorpheniramine blocking histamine receptors), another mechanism may involve the displacement of an inhibitor compound from its location on enzyme sites (e.g. pralidoxime reactivating cholinesterases that have been inhibited by some organophosphorus compounds) or there may be an effect brought about by changed toxicokinetics such as diminished uptake or increased excretion. These and other mechanisms of antagonism have important connotations in acute toxicology as they may form the basis of antidotes as well as being of theoretical and practical importance in relation to the events of multiple exposures.

Interactive effects can be specific and it is possible for closely related mixed exposures to produce different combination effects. For example, pralidoxime acts as an antagonist to chemicals that inhibit cholinesterases by phosphorylation but may actually enhance the acute toxicity of anticholinesterase agents that act by carbamylation of the enzymes[255,256]. In clinical toxicology effective treatment of acute intoxications may be dependent on awareness of this possibility.

Biometricians have devised procedures for the quantification and mathematical interpretation of interactive effects[170,253,254,257-269]. Interactive effects are of importance in environmental toxicology[247,270-273,677,678], the toxicology of therapeutic agents[238,274-281] and also in relation to the safe handling of chemicals[282-284] and quantification helps define the situation.

Investigations of possible interactive effects must take into account the sequence of the exposure (i.e. in a simple binary case, A before B; B before A or concurrent exposure to A and B). The magnitude of the exposures to each component A and B must always be considered[285]. Investigations generally include several combinations of exposure levels and the resulting data can be visualized graphically by means of isoboles[286].

Isoboles relate the relative exposure rates of the components (i.e. A and B) to the acute toxic responses (i.e. response due to A, response due to B and response due to [A + B]). The appearance of typical isoboles for binary combinations are illustrated in Figure 3.6. For interactive situations involving more than two

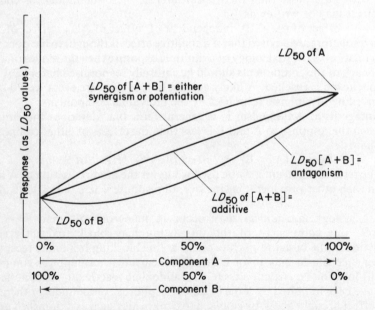

Fig. 3.6 A typical set of isoboles for binary mixtures (i.e. Two component toxicants designated A and B).

Table 3.3 Some interpretations of the index value (*V*) for interactive effects using formulae attributable to Clausing and Bieleke[285] and to Wysocka–Paruszewska et al[284]

	Values of V formulae (i) and (ii)	formula (iii)
Antagonism	<0.8	<0.7
Additive	0.8 to 1.5	0.7 to 1.3
more than Additive*	—	1.3 to 1.8
Potentiation or Synergism	>1.5	>1.8

*Considered by Wysocka–Paruszewska et al to be insufficiently large to be classified as potentiation or synergism

components it is possible to use isoboles[253,254,287,288] but these multi-dimensional graphs are best produced by computerized graphic techniques as they are very difficult to construct manually[617].

As an alternative to the use of isoboles there are some simple numeric methods that may be used in order to test for interactive effects. These formulae are used to generate index values (*V*) that may be interpreted by reference to Table 3.3.

The first two formulae, designated here as (i) and (ii), are attributable to Clausing and Bieleke[285] who considered that formula (ii) would give the more realistic results and that formula (i) could give erroneous findings if the dose–response line characteristics were shallow. Formula (iii) is attributable to Wysocka–Paruszewska and co-workers[284]:

$$V = \frac{\frac{1}{2}LD_{50}\,A \; + \; \frac{1}{2}LD_{50}\,B}{LD_{50}\,(A \; + \; B)} \tag{i}$$

$$V = \frac{LD_{25}\,A \; + \; LD_{25}\,B}{LD_{50}\,(A \; + \; B)} \tag{ii}$$

$$V = \frac{\text{expected } LD_{50} \text{ value of } (A \; + \; B)}{\text{observed } LD_{50} \text{ value of } (A \; + \; B)} \tag{iii}$$

A simple test that may be used to detect deviation from additive interaction depends on a reciprocal rule (iv) that can be applied to data[203]:

$$\frac{1}{\text{predicted } LD_{50}} = \frac{P_A}{LD_{50} \text{ of A}} + \frac{P_B}{LD_{50} \text{ of B}} \tag{iv}$$

when, P_A and P_B are the proportion of the dose contributed by each of the products A and B (*note*: in formula (iv) the proportions must be expressed as the percentage of each component divided by 100). Acute oral toxicities of 27 chemicals in 350 pair combinations were examined by Smyth, Jr. and co-workers[289] and they concluded that this reciprocal rule (alternatively called a harmonic mean formula) was a satisfactory test for additive effects.

Just as there can be species differences in response to acute intoxication by single products sometimes there can be species variation in interactive response to multiple exposures. Generally these species differences in response are quantitative rather than qualitative but this is not always the case. There are occasions when the effect of multiple exposure may be additive, or greater than additive, in some species and antagonistic in some other species[283] but this level of diversity is uncommon.

Clearly the influence of exposure to a chemical on subsequent exposure to the same chemical forms an essential part of the sub-acute toxicity investigations. The possibility of species specificity in relation to increased or decreased sensitivity to intoxiction must not be overlooked. Because of the extreme specificity associated with immuno-systems, the influence of sequential exposure in terms of anaphylactic responses are not likely to be detected in sub-acute toxicity tests.

3.4 Some Limitations of *in vivo* Models

Procedures for predicting acute toxicology have developed on the premise that there are physiological similarities between different species of vertebrates and that these similarities would be reflected in the responses of different animals to xenobiotics. Quite simply it has been assumed that predictive tests could be carried out in laboratory animals and the findings extrapolated to other, in this context, less readily available species. Now there is an increased realisation that species similarities are limited[182,185] and that these differences are fundamental to the science of toxicology[290-293].

Although some investigative acute toxicology is carried out in order to derive information that will be of benefit to species other than humans (i.e. wildlife and domesticated animals) the majority of investigations are intended to provide information on toxicity that can be extrapolated to man. This ability of man to use other animals on the basis of their apparent inferiority has been termed **speciesism**[294] and is the subject of controversy and debate. Just as there are few toxicologists who would deny that there are ethical and moral constraints on the use of animals for experimentation there are also ethical and moral as well as legal considerations that relate to the use of humans for experimental purposes[150,295]. The very nature of acute toxicology severely limits the utilization humans for this type of investigation and anthropomorphic consideration, as well as economics, have limited the use of non-human primates for this purpose. There is a consensus of informed opinion to support the opinion that non-human primates offer little advantage, and a lot of disadvantages, over other laboratory species in the context of acute toxicology[290,296-299]; hence the use of non-human primates is usually restricted to special cases where a defined need can be identified.

The majority of predictive mammalian acute and sub-acute toxicity tests are carried out using rodents (mostly rats and mice). Other mammalian species are less often used unless they have a particular relevance. The merits and short-comings of different species are dependent on the particular objectives of the investigation[291,300-314] and the extrapolation of findings from any species to another requires caution[292,293,648,650].

Because rodents are commonly used for predictive toxicity testing there is a common misconception that they are particularly good models of events that would occur if man were to be exposed to the same toxicants. There is no reason for assuming that rodents are going to mimic human response any more than any other species and the reason for the popularity of rodents is quite simply expediency. The reasons for the popularity of rodents can be summarized as follows:

(a) Some rodents (e.g. rats and mice) are easy to breed in substantial quantities.
(b) Laboratory bred rodents are easy to maintain.
(c) Rodents are cheap in relation to most other species.
(d) Defined rodent strains can be bred.
(e) Rodents exhibit minimum health problems because of ease with which specified pathogen free husbandry can be used.
(f) Rodent size minimizes the amount of product required for toxicity testing.
(g) It is generally easy to expose rodents to toxicants.
(h) Rodents are easy to observe for signs of intoxication.
(i) Rats and some, but not all other rodents are unable to exhibit a vomit reflex and therefore cannot void materials that are instilled into their stomachs[315].

In man, and some other animals, vomitting may be an important sign of intoxication as well as being a natural protective mechanism to void some of the toxicant before complete absorption occurs. This sign will not be observed in investigations using laboratory rats[315].

Substantial differences in species sensitivity to acute intoxication are not uncommon[154]. Sometimes these differences are particularly apparent across the different classes of the animal kingdom. Many types of fish, for example, are extremely sensitive to the lethal effects of natural pyrethrums and the synthetic pyrethroid insecticides whereas birds, in general, are remarkably resistant to intoxication by these same pesticides[667].

With some products there are substantial differences in sensitivity to acute intoxication even within a class of animals. Because of differences in absorption, metabolism and distribution of the organophosphorus compound chlorfenvinphos and also because of differences in the relative sensitivities of the brain cholinesterases to inhibition by this compound, there are at least three orders of magnitude difference between the susceptibilities of rats and dogs to acute intoxication[316]. Species differences in sensitivity to other organophosphorus compounds have been observed[693]. Swine are remarkably insensitive to the acute toxic effects of the *Clostridium botulinium* toxins[317] but, compared with many other mammals, swine are very sensitive to intoxication by sodium chloride[318].

Every predictive toxicology investigation should include a thorough study of all that occurs as a result of the exposure[293,319,320]. It is essential that the validity of the test model for the particular route of exposure is checked at the outset of the investigation[268,321-325]. It is never valid to categorize animals, including man, as homogenous entities for there are innumerable variables within any species.

There are substantial physiological variations between individuals within a species and part of these variations is of genetic origin[631]. For example, in man it has been found that there are ethnic differences in the permeability of erythrocytes to sodium ions[326] and it is likely that even this apparently small variation may have implications in the observed ethnic differences in sensitivity to some toxicants. With laboratory animals destined for use in investigative toxicology, it is usual to minimize species variability by controlled breeding; this is clearly impossible for humans or for the animal population at large.

Under controlled conditions many animals can be categorized into defined strains or breeds. Humans can only be categorized on the much wider basis of ethnic groups. Ethnic grouping includes very diverse physiological character-istics. The study of pharmacological and toxicological responses associated with differences in strain, breed or ethnic characteristics is referred to by the general term **pharmacogenetics**[327,631].

There are many examples of differences in acute and sub-acute toxicity being linked to genetic characteristics[327-334,631]. A few illustrative examples include the marked differences in sensitivity of different strains of laboratory mice to fluor-enylacetamide[335], BHC[336] and 2,3,7,8-tetrachloro-dibenzo-*p*-dioxin[337]. A thera-peutically important example of ethnic differences in sensitivity to the toxic effects of chemicals is provided by the clinically significant, haemolysis that occurs in a high proportion of Negro people, but very rarely in Caucasians, when they are exposed to some anti-malarial drugs (e.g. primaquine) or many of the therapeutic sulphonamides and sulphones; this ethnic difference in sensitivity is associated with a deficiency of the enzyme glucose-6-phosphate dehydrogenase in a substantial proportion of members of the negroid races whereas the enzyme is rarely deficient in other ethnic groups[631].

Even with knowledge of pharmacogenetic background it is not always possible to predict with certainty the responses that will occur at the individual level[631,639]. In any population there are likely to be individuals who will exhibit idiosyncratic responses even at toxicant exposure levels that are tolerated by others in the same population[338,339,639]. Sometimes idiosyncratic anaphylactic reactions occur in response to very small toxicant exposures. Often the exposure is much less than the expected toxic level and, at present there is no meaningful technique available for predicting idiosyncratic reactions[639].

Because of the close interrelationship that exists between age and growth caution is necessary when distinguishing effects that are manifestations of body size from those that are associated with other aspects of the aging process[629,686]. In clinical medicine it is common practice to calculate the dosage of therapeutic agents for children on the basis of one of several posological formulae that take into account either age or physical dimensions of the child[340] but there is no simple correlation between age and sensitivity to acute intoxication by most products[341,686]. To obtain any relationship between age and toxic dose levels it is necessary to consider every toxicant and each species individually[342,343].

An age profile that may be applied when considering all animal species can be set out as follows:

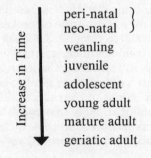

The actual time span for this profile varies between species so that, for example, with the laboratory rat the whole profile is completed in about 2 or 3 years whereas in man it takes about 70 to 80 years. Aging is, of course, a continuous process and the sub-divisions shown in the profile do not represent any sharp dividing lines in the life process but rather they are a sequence of gradual transitions. Even if it is assumed that all animals remain entirely healthy for the whole life-span, clearly a false assumption, the number of changes that occur in the overall physiology with the passage of time are numerous and each change influences responses in acute intoxication[180,342-345,686].

Many of the physiological changes that occur during the aging process are well defined but there are some that still remain controversial. The blood–brain barrier exemplifies this uncertainty; the function of the blood–brain barrier is critically important in the toxicokinetics of some chemicals but there are uncertainties as to whether the blood–brain barrier is fully functional in some young mammals and this may influence the apparent age dependent toxico-kinetics observed with some chemicals in different species.

In the age profile scheme, the terms peri-natal and neo-natal are shown bracketed together. The term peri-natal is associated with part of the time that the offspring is *in utero* and part immediately after birth; Khera and Clegg[346] defined peri-natal, in respect of humans, as the time interval from the termination of organogenesis until four weeks *post partum*. Conventionally the toxic effects of chemicals *ante partum* are not considered as being part of the science of acute toxicology but are studied under the categories of reproductive toxicology and teratology; acute toxicology is considered to be appropriate from the neo-natal stage of development onwards and that convention is followed here.

Neo-natal animals are susceptible to acute intoxication in various ways[626-628]. Translocation of toxicants from the mother to the neo-nate via the milk can be a problem and there are some toxicants (e.g. iodides) that are concentrated in milk to levels that exceed the maternal plasma concentration; some commonly used drugs (e.g. some barbiturates and diazepam) and some slowly metabolized lipophilic pesticides (e.g. dieldrin, DDT, etc.) can translocate in milk from exposed mothers and cause acute intoxication in their neo-natal offspring[696,697].

Adventitious exposure of neo-natal animals occurs on many occasions. Domesticated animals have been intoxicated because of the use of wood that has been treated with preservatives, such as dieldrin or pentachlorophenols, to produce the saw-dust and wood shavings used in animal husbandry[243,244]. Human neo-nates have been exposed to baby-care products containing toxic chemicals[347], such as boron derivatives[348-349] or hexachlorophane[350-351] with tragic consequences.

Neo-nates are always potentially at risk if they are exposed to therapeutic medication[347,352-355] and particular care must be exercised in determining the appropriate dosage regimen. On a body weight basis it is wrong to assume that neo-natal animals are always more susceptible to acute intoxication than older animals[356]. It has been observed that neo-natal animals are generally less sensitive to intoxication by organochlorine pesticides than are older animals of the same species[357,358] whereas the opposite holds for intoxication by organo-phosphorus anticholinesterase compounds[359,360].

Once animals achieve weanling status they undergo physiological changes that are associated with transition from a diet of mothers' milk to solid foods. The hepatic enzyme systems become more active and, with the exception of sexual development, the animals become more physiologically mature at the weanling stage of development but for acute intoxication the pattern of sensitivity is complex. One group of investigators[353] found that sixteen out of thirty diverse compounds tested were more toxic to new-born rats than to adult rats but they also found that new-born rats were less susceptible to intoxication by central nervous system stimulants than were the adult rats. Other investigators demonstrated that the central nervous system depressant morphine is significantly more acutely toxic to immature rats than it is to adult rats[361]. With a large number of organophosphorus compounds and carbamates that have been examined in both weanling and adult rats it has been reported that only one compound had a lower LD_{50} value (i.e. was more acutely toxic) in adults than it was in weanling animals[357]. Clearly there is not one factor that explains all of the differences in sensitivity to acute intoxication experienced with these various age groups. Undoubtedly the activities of the hepatic microsomal enzyme systems influence the acute toxicity associated with some classes of chemicals[250], for example, investigations of the acute intraperitoneal toxicity of carbon disulfide in rats ranging in age from 1 day (LD_{50} value 583 mg kg^{-1}) to 20 days (LD_{50} value 1545 mg kg^{-1}) revealed that the effects of the carbon disulphide on the mixed function oxidase system and the conversion of carbon disulphide to a covalently binding, sulphur-containing, biotransformation product varied with the age of the rats[674]. Other toxicokinetic differences are also very important[352-361].

Differences in sensitivity to acute intoxication by physiological as well as xenobiotic chemicals have been observed in studies with neo-nates in relation to adult animals[626-628]. Adult mice are, for example, significantly more sensitive to acute intoxication by adrenaline and nor-adrenaline than are neo-natal mice[362].

In humans an important example of age related difference in sensitivity to acute intoxication has been experienced with some therapeutic iron products. Until the 1970's the incidence of acute iron poisoning in children was very common and iron appeared high on the lists of causative agents in reported cases of acute poisoning in the USA and several other countries[363,364] whereas acute iron intoxication among adults is rare and most iron compounds that are used therapeutically are well tolerated by adults. Diminution in the incidence of acute iron intoxication in children has been achieved by recognition of the problem followed by appropriate remedial and preventative action, and cannot be attributed to changes in the sensitivity to this group of chemicals.

Most routine predictive acute and sub-acute toxicity testing utilizes 'young adult' animals. The specification of 'young adult' varies considerably and requires careful definition in relation to the interpretation of data obtained from an investigation. Using laboratory rats to illustrate this point; some investigators define the chosen animals by selection of a weight range (say 150 to 250 grams) whereas others select from an age range (perhaps 8 to 12 weeks old). Even on the basis of a defined population the age–weight relationship is not linear and that there can be real differences in the ratios for males and females. Population averages mask important individual differences and this masking is much more apparent with some species, not least humans, than it is with laboratory rodents.

Mature and geriatric animals exhibit varying degrees of ablation of physiological function[629,686]. Functional efficiency of the brain can alter sensitivity to centrally acting toxicants[365] and hepatic microsomal enzyme activities diminish with old age and this can influence sensitivity to acute intoxication[366]. The whole pattern of toxicokinetics for many products changes with the aging process and it is not possible to single out a universal model that includes all of the numerous variables[367-369,629,686]. An endorsement of the complexity of this lack of age related uniformity in acute toxicology is found with the variable patterns of response associated with some toxicants in different species[370]. The acute toxicity of the alkaloid atropine illustrates this point, viz atropine is more toxic to immature dogs than to adult dogs but the opposite sensitivity applies to rabbits and there is uniformity of sensitivity to atropine in rats of all ages.

Fatalities have occurred in elderly people being treated with some of the non-steroidal anti-inflammatory drugs because of the failure to recognize the longer metabolic half-life of these drugs in older people than in young adults; this despite the fact that elderly people are more likely to suffer from the type of inflammatory disease that would benefit from these drugs more than most younger people[688].

It is not only in mammals that sensitivity to acute intoxication is influenced by age. Age-linked sensitivity to the acute toxic properties of some products has been found to occur in fish[371] and also birds[372]; it is probable that the same phenomenon occurs in amphibians and reptiles but there is not sufficient definitive data available to ensure certainty.

Most of the differences in susceptibility to acute intoxication that are attributable to the sex of the exposed animals are associated with quantitative, rather than qualitative, differences in the physiology and this accounts for the lack of consistency found for male and female animals of different species or even different strains of the same species. Toxicokinetics can, for example, be influenced by sex related differences in body fluid or body fat distribution or the differences in the activities of enzymes that are present in both sexes.

Many products are equi-toxic to animals of both sexes and some are more toxic to one sex than the other. There is no simple rule relating sensitivity to sex and sometimes it is found that the ratio of sensitivity is different in different species and sometimes marked differences are found with different strains of the same species[373,374].

For products that are not equi-toxic to animals of both sexes it is more common to find that females are more susceptible than males and experience has shown that this is particularly the case with laboratory rats[375]. However, there are many exceptions for which male rats are more sensitive than females such as the anticoagulant hydroxycoumarin derivatives and several pesticides (e.g. aldrin, chlordane, methyl parathion, etc)[375]. An example of inconsistency in the sex related sensitivity is found with the organophosphorus compound, mevinphos, which is more toxic to female rats than to male rats[375] but the opposite ratio is true for the Mongolian gerbil[376].

Sex related differences in sensitivity to acute intoxication are sometimes due to the relative activities of hepatic microsomal enzymes in each sex[377-379]. Investigations into the influence of hepatic microsomal enzyme activities in rats, mice and rabbits has provided evidence that observed differences in the sensitivities of these three types of animals and, very importantly, the differences in sensitivities found in males and females of each species can be correlated with these enzyme activities[380]. The sensitivity of some animals to intoxication may be significantly changed during pregnancy[654]. For example, the clearance of the analgesic drug paracetamol is about twice the rate in pregnant women that it is in other women. This difference with paracetamol can be explained by the rapid elimination of the glucuronide and glutathione-derived conjugates during pregnancy[630].

An example of a species specific, sex related sensitivity to the acute toxic properties of a chemical is found with the chemotherapeutic agent, oxamniquine, which has been shown to be more toxic to laboratory rats than to several other species of laboratory animals and also it has been demonstrated that there is a sex-linked differential in the acute toxicity of oxamniquine to rats. The investigators[381] have suggested that hepatic metabolizing enzymes may be responsible for these species and sex related differences in sensitivity to intoxication by oxamniquine, hepatotoxicity being peculiar to the rats but not the other species exposed to this compound.

An objective of modern laboratory animal technology is to minimize stress in experimental animals and yet the data obtained from these minimal stress conditions is used to predict acute toxicity in man, or other animals, living in stressful conditions.

Physiological stress may be associated with many different causes and influences. Some of the important stress factors influencing acute and sub-acute intoxication are:

(i) **Nutritional Status**. Predictive acute toxicity testing, at least by the oral route, is usually carried out using animals that have not had access to food for several hours before the exposure[620]. For some other routes of exposure food may be withheld during the actual exposure period (e.g. some inhalation tests). The investigation has to take into account the influence of gastro-intestinal contents on toxicokinetics[240,382,619] and also the fact that withholding food can induce changes in the physiology and biochemistry of animals[383-385,684]. If the withholding of food is continued for too long (i.e. longer than the 18 hours generally used for peroral acute toxicity tests) then the physiological and biochemical changes that occur will influence the toxicokinetics of any product[386,387]. The magnitude and nature of change in sensitivity to acute intoxication will be influenced by the species and possibly the sex of the animal[388]. Inadequate diets and chronic malnutrition are commonplace among animals including man. Malnutrition sometimes causes animals to ingest toxic materials in their search for foodstuff among inappropriate sources. Malnutrition is often associated with diseases and there is an increased risk of acute intoxication by drugs used to treat the ailment[389,390,684].

Deficiency of any of the nutritional dietary components, over a period of time, may change the response of animals to xenobiotics[389-392,684] and the nature of the changes, in respect of acute and sub-acute toxicology, can be very variable[619].

Dietary excesses, like deficiencies, can influence responses to xenobiotics but generally this is more apparent in relation to chronic rather than acute or sub-acute exposure[389,392,684]. For example, protein intake, whether above or below the nutritional normal requirement, has been shown to have a profound effect on the acute toxicities of several chemicals[393].

(ii) **Biological Rhythms**. Chronobiologists have devised a detailed nomenclature to describe the time intervals associated with biological rhythms[394-396]; but the following attenuated form of the nomenclature[397] is adequate for use in acute toxicology:

Title	Time Period
ultradian	more than one day
circadian	one day
infradian	less than one day

The extraneous factors that act as markers for biological rhythms are called **zeitgebers** (from the German meaning, 'time donor') and the two most important zeitgebers in acute toxicology are ambient temperature and the periodicity of light and darkness[398]. Abolition of any zeitgeber may not entirely change the physiological sequence that it normally triggers and physiological adaptation to changes in any zeitgeber is often achieved rapidly.

During acute and sub-acute toxicity testing it is usual for laboratory animals to be maintained under thermoneutral conditions and generally the lighting is time-controlled to provide defined periods of light and darkness. Rodents are at their most active in the dark and it is during the period of darkness that important signs of intoxication may occur and are most likely to be missed by investigators. If a sub-acute exposure investigation is being carried out with the toxicant being administered in the food or drinking water, it must be remembered that animals do not eat all of the time and that their feeding habits are often linked to the light and darkness sequence; rodents eat most during the periods of darkness when they are at their most active state, some other animals prefer to eat during the periods of light and to sleep in the dark.

It is not possible to establish any single factor as being responsible for all of the biological rhythm effects that occur in toxicology and some examples illustrate this point:

Mice exhibit circadian rhythm in their response to some convulsants[399] and it has been demonstrated that the acute toxicity of nikethamide, a cerebral stimulant, varies with the time of day when it is administered by the subcutaneous route[400,401].

The hepatotoxicity associated with tetrachloromethane and the nephrotoxicity caused by mercuric chloride are both maximal at the active times of the day and it has been suggested that these effects are related to the circadian biochemical activities of the liver and kidneys[402]. There is considerable published support for the idea that rhythmic patterns of response are associated with rhythms in the biochemistry of each animal[403-408]. Circadian variations in the activities of hepatic enzymes can be influenced by food intake[409,410] and this, in turn, may be influenced by the sex of the animal. There is some evidence suggesting that there are endocrine factors involved in the control mechanism of the various enzyme activities at different periods in the circadian cycle[411,414].

In addition to the metabolizing enzyme systems there are other factors that may have a significant role in the rhythmic changes associated with response to intoxication. These other factors include changes in absorption, distribution and the receptor sites[411-413], changes in hormonal activity[414] and immunological factors[675].

(iii) Physiological stress involves perturbation of the endocrine balance associated with the pituitary–adrenal axis and this perturbation may result from many factors. Selective ablation of the pituitary–adrenal axis, by either adrenalectomy or hypophysectomy, markedly alters responses to many xenobiotic chemicals. Mostly the changes are quantitative rather than qualitative and the magnitude of the influence associated with these methods of ablation differs considerably between different species and may even differ between the sexes of a species[415].

Some toxicants are capable of interfering with the function of the pituitary–adrenal axis and these may induce a stress related symptomatology[416,417]. One sequence of stress that can be important in the toxicokinetics associated with acute exposure is change in the permeability of the blood-brain-barrier[418] and the significance of the blood-brain-barrier in the distribution of centrally acting toxicants may be very great indeed.

Stress occurs as a result of numerous different stimuli and investigators must recognize the stress inducing nature of seemingly minor details of experimental procedures[419].

Some laboratory animals, particularly rodents, are gregarious and the relative merits of carrying out experiments with isolated (i.e. one animal in a cage) or aggregated (i.e. more than one animal per cage) animals in toxicity testing is problematic. Although the animals are gregarious there is also a strong tendency for dominance to be part of communal living thus animals that have been affected by a toxicant are likely to be prevented from eating or drinking, by other unaffected, or less affected, animals in the same cage. Even more apparent with some species is cannabalism and any weakened animal is likely to be attacked and eaten by other animals in the same cage. For these reasons, coupled with ease of observations, it is generally more satisfactory from the practical but not the theoretical point-of-view, to have each animal isolated[420]. The stress effects of isolation on gregarious animals can be great and this does not only apply to the status of the animals during the time that they are exposed to the toxicant but it has been shown that isolation of aggregation before exposure can also influence the outcome of subsequent exposure to toxicants[420-422].

Investigations of the acute toxicology of chemicals that act on the central nervous system have revealed that the responses to the same product under identical conditions, with the sole exception that some animals were isolated and others aggregated, can be quantitatively very different from each other[235,236,422]. Both the CNS stimulant amphetamine[423] and the CNS depressant morphine[424] are markedly more acutely toxic to aggregated mice than they are to isolated mice.

Variable degrees of physiological stress are introduced into any acute or sub-acute toxicity investigation by the technical competence of the investigators and it is an essential objective that unwanted and uncontrolled physiological stress must be kept to a minimum.

(iv) Environmental temperature markedly affects the sensitivity of animals to many toxicants but the majority of investigations in predictive acute toxicology are carried out with the animals maintained in conditions that are within the thermoneutral range. Sometimes the need for studies at elevated or lowered temperatures is recognized. From the data that are available it is clear that there is no simple relationship between ambient temperature and sensitivity to acute intoxication and the influence on each toxicant has to be considered individually.

Some published examples of the influence of ambient temperature include the fact that rats maintained in a cold environment (4°C ± 1°C) were found to be between 1000 and 10 000 times more sensitive to acute intoxication by isoprenaline than those maintained in thermoneutral conditions[425]. Other investigators[426] maintained groups of mice at each of three different ambient temperatures for 24 hours before and then during and after exposure to one of three diverse toxicants, pentobarbitone, adrenaline and acetylcholine; of these three compounds it was found that only pentobarbitone was less toxic at an elevated temperature than at the thermoneutral temperature and the same compound was more toxic at a lower than thermoneutral temperature whereas the other two products, adrenaline and acetylcholine, were more toxic at lowered and elevated temperatures than they were at the thermoneutral temperature (See Table 3.4).

From the limited amount of definitive data that are available it may be concluded that at temperatures below the thermoneutral range it is fairly common to find that either increased or decreased sensitivity to acute intoxication occurs whereas with ambient temperatures above the thermoneutral range it is rare to find diminished sensitivity but common to find increased sensitivity to acute intoxication.[426-430].

Prolonged exposure of animals to extremes of ambient temperature can affect sensitivity to intoxication by some products[431] and this may result from changes in the associated toxicokinetics[432].

Physiological thermoregulatory mechanisms are susceptible to interference by some toxicants[433]. The best known examples of fatal human intoxication occurring as a result of interference with thermal homeostasis occurred following exposure to two chemicals, 3,5-dinitro-*o*-cresol and 2,4-dinitrophenol. Both of these phenolic derivatives were used in armaments manufacture during the 1914–1918 World War and then subsequently they were used as pesticides and also as drugs to aid slimming. In the mammalian body

Table 3.4 The acute intraperitoneal LD_{50} values for three toxicants in mice (ICR/JCC strain) maintained at each of three different ambient temperatures. (Data published by Yamauchi et al[426])

Toxicant	LD_{50} value (mg kg^{-1})		
	20 °C	25 °C	35 °C
Pentobarbital	57	101	135
Adrenaline	5.0	14.6	7.4
Acetylcholine	178	216	166

*Confidence limits not quoted by Investigators

3,5-dinitro-*o*-cresol and 2,4-dinitrophenol are potent uncouplers of the mitochondrial oxidative phosphorylation process and this uncoupling action allows the generation of metabolic heat in excess of the heat-dissipating ability of the body. These two chemicals have caused numerous human deaths as a result of both deliberate and accidental exposures[689].

When alphachloralose is used as a rodenticide it is more effective at lower temperatures than at the thermoneutral or elevated temperatures[434]. A practical implication of this is that heat exchange between the exposed animals and the environment is related to body surface area and this, in turn, means that small rodents, such as mice, are more sensitive to alphachloralose intoxication than are large rodents[435]. Although other, larger, animals have been affected by ingesting rodenticide bait containing alphachloralose[436] it is generally less toxic to larger animals than it is to smaller animals and this is an important safeguard in its use.

Uptake of toxicants by any route may be influenced by ambient temperature but this is generally most apparent in relation to inhalation exposure[437,438] and percutaneous absorption[239] and this must be treated as an important variable when considering acute or sub-acute toxicity. The sensitivity of poikilothermal animals to acute intoxication by chemicals can be influenced by ambient temperature[154] but there are little data available on poikilothermal species, other than fish, in this context[439,440]. Even among different species of fish the influence of ambient temperature varies[441,442] and it is not realistic to generalize about the acute toxicities of chemicals to fish in relation to ambient temperature.

Atmospheric humidity is an ambient climatic variable. Just as the majority of predictive acute toxicity tests are carried out with the exposed animals maintained in an environment that is in the thermoneutral range it is also usual to control the relative humidity of the atmosphere at a comfortable level. One of the few published investigations into the effects of ambient relative humidity on acute toxicity set out to correlate ambient relative humidity measurements with variations in acute intraperitoneal toxicity of nicotine bitartrate in rats. The investigators[428] found that at the higher humidities the physiological heat exchange mechanism of the rats failed and that there was a correlation between increases in relative humidity and decreases in LD_{50} values.

Because of species differences in ability to sweat it is certain that the influence of ambient humidity on acute toxicity will be affected by the particular target species. With the knowledge that many drugs, pesticides and other chemicals are used in tropical climates and also in climates that are sub-temperate there is a need for further research into the relationships that exist between ambient conditions and toxic responses[443,444].

There are not many other environmental factors that seriously influence the acute toxicities of products in terrestial vertebrates. In aquatic environments ambient conditions can influence acute toxicities to aquatic vertebrates. In addition to interactive effects of toxicants with other pollutants, the three most important influences are the pH, the hardness and the oxygen tension associated with the water in which the exposure occurs[445] and their effects will vary with the nature of the toxicant and the particular target species.

3.5 Tolerance

Tolerance may be considered as a special case of interactive effect (Section 3.3) in which auto-desensitization to acute intoxication occurs. Desensitization may result from previous prolonged or repeated exposure to the toxicant or, occasionally, to a similar product. Tolerance cannot be induced by all toxic substances. Where tolerance has developed in a target it is generally found that the relevant detoxifying enzyme systems have been stimulated to greater than normal activity and there may also be changes in the excretory mechanisms facilitating removal of the toxicant.

Auto-desensitization is a phenomenon often observed in people who have become addicted to narcotics; these people are often able to withstand single doses of one particular drug that would be lethal to normal, non-addicted, subjects. Tolerance to some chemicals may develop as an inherited characteristic and this can be of biological and economic significance with some toxic chemicals used for vertebrate pest control[446] and studies of this type of tolerance fall into the category of pharmacogenetics[327,328,631].

Tolerance to acute toxic effects of chemicals is not restricted to higher vertebrates but is also known to occur in fish[447] and amphibians[439], this is an important attribute for the survival of some species in situations of environmental contamination. Tolerance development is often detectable in predictive sub-acute toxicity testing and the investigations have to be designed to reveal this possibility. Clearly tolerance is likely to be related to the ability of exposed animals to adapt to metabolic changes and this may not be common to all species for any particular toxicant. To investigate the development of tolerance it is generally necessary to undertake detailed metabolism and toxicokinetic studies.

4

Reduction, Refinement and Replacement

Objection to the use of living animals for research purposes is not new but the level of awareness of the moral and ethical considerations associated with this contentious subject is now greater than ever before[294,448-453]. The majority of toxicologists are committed to the principles of the '3R's'[457]. The '3R's' are defined as: **replacement** of animal experimentation whenever possible and including replacement of outmoded methodology by the introduction of **refinements**; from these two achievements there will be a **reduction** in the number of living animals used in experiments. Total replacement of *in vivo* animal experimentation in acute and sub-acute investigative toxicology is a laudable long-term objective with little chance of total achievement, at least in the foreseeable future, whereas reduction in the number of animals used can readily be achieved. In this context **refinement** can be defined as reduction of suffering to an absolute minimum including, if possible, total elimination[638]. Care is necessary if objectives are not to become confused, in other words, it is necessary to question whether a reduction in the numbers of animals used is justifiable if the experimental design or procedure then necessitates an increased level of suffering in the smaller number of exposed animals.

Predictive acute toxicology has been singled out as being one of the most severe procedures forming part of the toxicological assessment of products[155]. There have been many statements of intent about the reduction in the numbers of animals that should be used in predictive acute toxicology[155,163,454,455]. Alternatives to the use of living animals for predictive acute and sub-acute toxicology fall into two distinct categories. Firstly, there are methods requiring materials of animal origin; these often necessitate the death of some animals, albeit painlessly, to provide the necessary tissues, organs, enzymes, etc. Secondly, there are methods independent of animal derived materials. Many of the areas of endeavour relevant to replacement, refinment and reduction in acute and sub-acute toxicology are being investigated in various international centres; a summary of the state of knowledge follows:

4.1 Cell and Tissue Culture Methods

The culture *in vitro* of cells and tissues is not a new idea but the techniques available for the maintenance and perpetuation of the cells and tissues have been greatly improved[621].

Cultures of cells and tissues are only able to respond to the direct effects of toxicants acting directly at the cellular level and they are not able to respond to multi-stage pharmacological action[670,671]. Biochemical processes that involve other organs or systems when exposure occurs *in vivo* (e.g. toxification or detoxification) cannot be anticipated from this type of *in vitro* investigation other than the limited investigation of *in vitro* metabolism by isolated enzyme systems (e.g. fractionated liver homogenates) used in association with culture method.

Cells and tissues exposed to toxicants *in vitro* are not capable of demonstrating any of the symptomatology that is associated with acute intoxication[456-465] and a further limitation of the *in vitro* tissue or organ methodology is its inability to mimic the *in vivo* toxicokinetic influences that are characterized by bioavailability of the toxicant[670,671].

For those classes of chemicals exhibiting toxicity characteristics that are known to relate to specific target organs there can be some merit in carrying out investigations by using cultured preparations of the known target system[464-469]. Genetic differences in sensitivity of response can be detected using culture systems[470] but confidence in the methodology has been diminished by the finding that the very highly toxic compound, 2,3,7,8-tetrachlorodibenzo-*p*-dioxin, with its established organ directed toxicology[644] has given results that are not consistent with *in vivo* experience in detailed investigations with cultured cells[471]. Cell, tissue and organ culture research is being carried out on an extensive scale throughout the World and it remains to be seen whether this will have a major impact on the need for predictive acute toxicity tests carried out *in vivo*[460,465,466,468,469,472-474,690,691]. At this time, isolated hepatocytes in culture are attracting a lot of interest as a possible screening model for acute cytotoxic effects[692] but it is not anticipated that isolated hepatocytes will provide a universal screening method for all forms of acute toxic effect[475].

4.2 Techniques using Isolated Biomolecules

Some products are toxic because of their ability to interact with biomolecules rather than with cells. Techniques of modern biochemistry allow the isolation and physico–chemical definition of many biomolecules and it is often technically easy to study the interactions between these molecules and various xenobiotics *in vitro*. Studies with isolated biomolecules are useful as an aid to the interpretation of mode of action of toxicants but correlation with *in vivo* acute toxicology is generally limited.

An example of the isolated biomolecule approach is found with derivatives of fluoroacetic acid. It is demonstrable, *in vitro*, that these compounds block the physiological citric acid cycle[478] (see Figure 4.1) and because of this property they are highly toxic to vertebrate animals[476-478]. Due to the acute toxicity of some of these fluorocompounds they have been widely used for killing vermin[477] and they have been implicated in numerous other acute intoxications but the use of *in vitro* techniques has not been successful in predicting the wide disparity in sensitivity to intoxication found with different species[477], in other words, the *in vivo* toxicokinetics may profoundly affect the outcome of exposure.

Another example of this approach is found with the cholinesterase enzymes. These enzymes have been researched in great detail and cholinesterases are very amenable to studies using both *in vivo* and *in vitro* methodology. Many carbamates[480] and organophosphorus compounds[479] are inhibitors of the various cholinesterase activities both *in vivo* and *in vitro*; important

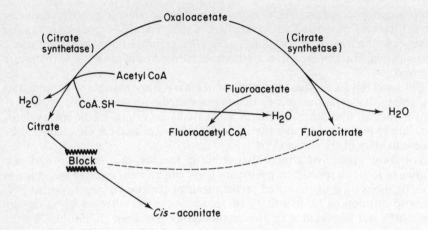

Fig. 4.1   Fluoroacetate interference with the physiological citric acid cycle.

information about the nature of the enzyme inhibition can be derived from reversibility studies including the use of reactivators[481-483]. Data establishing differences in the activities of cholinesterases from various physiological locations within individuals and differences in the characteristics of these enzymes found in different species are plentiful[484-486,693] but very little correlation between the inhibition of cholinesterases *in vivo* and the inhibition of these enzymes *in vitro* has been established[487,693].

Reasons for lack of correlation between the acute toxicity and *in vitro* enzyme interactions include the toxicokinetics that are a function of exposed whole living targets[316]. For example, thiono-organophosphates are weak inhibitors of cholinesterases whereas the corresponding thiolo-form of these phosphates are potent inhibitors, consequently the thiolo-phosphates are very much more toxic to vertebrates[488,489]. The acute toxicities of thiono-organophosphates to animals results from *in vivo* toxification to the thiolo-form and this toxification does not occur *in vitro*. The efficiency of toxification varies among different species and this accounts for quite marked differences in the susceptibility of different species to intoxication by these compounds[489,490]. To illustrate these differences, data for the acute toxicities of two thiono-organophosphorus compounds, malathion and sumithion, are shown together with the corresponding data for their thiolo-analogues in Table 4.1.

Inhibitors of monoamine oxidase are another group of chemicals that exert pharmacological effects because of a specific enzyme inhibitory property. Some correlation between this enzyme inhibitory property measured *in vitro* and the acute toxicology associated with individual chemicals in this group has been established[491].

Toxicokinetic characteristics of the cytotoxic drug cytosine arabinoside have been cited as an example of correlation between *in vitro* and *in vivo* species dependent metabolism[293]. The distribution and specific activities of pyrimidine nucleoside deaminase, the enzyme required to convert cytosine arabinoside to uracil arabinoside, is a variable between species; by investigating, this enzyme from different sources *in vitro* and then relating the information to cytotoxicity *in vivo* good correlations have been deduced[293].

Table 4.1 The acute toxicities of some chemically related pairs of organophosphorus compounds

(a) Compounds administered, as solutions, by intraperitoneal injection to rabits.

(Data from Cheymol *et al*[488])

LD_{50} in mg kg^{-1} (95% Confidence Limits)	

R_1
   \ |
     P – O – C –
   /   \\\ |
R_2 S
	R_1
	   \ |
	     P – S – C –
	   / \\\ |
	R_2 O

Malathion 1280 (1090 – 1500)	isoMalathion 72 (69 – 73)
Sumithion 960 (815 – 1132)	isoSumithion 150 (127 – 177)

(b) Undiluted compounds administered to rats by intragastric intubation. (Data from Lovell[487])

Approximate LD_{50} in mg kg^{-1}	
Malathion 2600	isoMalathion 88

The effects of toxicants on isolated biomolecules form an important part of overall investigations into mechanisms of pharmacological and toxic actions but this approach alone does not constitute an adequate substitute for *in vivo* acute toxicity testing.

4.3 Avian Embryos

Some investigators consider avian embryos to be reasonable models of vertebrate physiological systems for investigative purposes. These embryos are readily accessible, easy to manipulate and are free from some of the characteristics of the sentient free-living vertebrate animals commonly used in predictive acute toxicity testing.

Although avian embryos possess more of the functional physiological characteristics of free-living vertebrate animal than are found with isolated cells or organs (Section 4.1) the similarities are very limited. Avian embryos have been used to investigate the teratological potential of chemicals[492] and it was from a group of teratologists, who were working with avian embryos, that the first publication of the use of these organisms for predicting acute toxic potential originated[493] and the overlap of interest in this model for both types of investigation is obvious[494,495].

Techniques for assessing toxicity by means of avian embryos are generally dependent on the toxicant being injected into the yolk sacs of several fertilized eggs followed by incubation to allow any surviving embryos to develop. If an embryo does not develop death is attributed to the toxicity of the injected chemical although any investigation includes control groups of eggs (i.e. fertilized eggs that have been injected with the vehicle only) in order to check on viability of the eggs under the conditions of the test.

There are several important practical points about methodology using avian embryos. Firstly, it is necessary to distribute the toxicant evenly in the contents of the yolk sac and with some chemicals it is difficult to achieve homogeneous distribution and this may cause some developing embryos to be exposed to more or less than the anticipated dose of toxicant.

Distribution of any toxicant within an egg is affected by its lipophilicity[496]; in general lipophilic toxicants distribute more evenly in the egg yolk than lipophobic chemicals. Secondly, even if it is assumed that distribution of the toxicant within the yolk is uniform there is no obvious relationship between the exposure experienced by the embryo and the dose level that would equate to exposure in free living animals. Despite this lack of correlation of exposure levels it has been reported that avian embryo methods are capable of a high level of prediction for the acute toxicity rating of some mycotoxins when avian embryos mortalities are compared with that data obtained using rats as the test species[497].

Most of these investigations are carried out on the fertilized eggs of domestic fowl because of easy availability. The eggs of ducks have also been used and some investigators have reported that results with these eggs have given more reliable data than chicken eggs although no explanation of the difference between the two is known[498]. These same investigators also found a good correlation between results obtained with avian eggs and LD_{50} values obtained using rats with some, but not all, of the chemicals tested by both methods[498].

Although the idea of using avian embryos for predictive acute toxicology has some attractions, it is likely that this technique will only provide a scale of relative acute toxicities for a series of chemicals rather than absolute values for individual products. Avian egg methods cannot provide information on symptomatology.

4.4 Models that use isolated Organs

Isolated organs have been used in experimental pharmacology for a long time and there are occasions when this approach to the mechanism of action, at the organ level, can be helpful to the understanding of toxic properties. It is in the investigation of toxicodynamics that isolated organ techniques have proved most useful.

4.4.1 Gastro-intestinal absorption

By the use of isolated lengths of the alimentary tract, either removed from freshly killed animals or left *in situ* in fresh cadavers, it is technically easy to measure uptake of toxicants through portions of the digestive tract into perfusates[499-505]. From analyses of the perfusates deductions can be made about the physico–chemical characteristics of the toxicant and these data can be related to uptake. This approach has proved particularly useful for comparing the alimentary uptakes of members of various homologous series[503,504]. This methodology may also be used for comparing the bioavailability of toxicants, when presented in different formulations but these techniques only relate to penetration through a membrane system and the same organs behave differently *in vivo*.

4.4.2 Percutaneous absorption

For the purpose of *in vitro* absorption studies skin has often been considered as though it is a simple membrane system and the mathematical principles that underlie membrane physics have been used frequently to explain the percutaneous absorption characteristics of toxicants[506-510].

Because of the ease of availability of human skin for *in vitro* experimentation the problems associated with extrapolation of data from one species to another need not arise. However, there are significant differences in the pentrability of human skin obtained from different anatomical locations, and there are likely to be marked differences between absorption characteristics when measured using small pieces of skin *in vitro* from those that would be experienced with the same toxicant in contact with larger areas of skin *in vivo*[239,506,507].

Without the need to undertake any experimentation it is sometimes possible to predict, from known physico-chemical characteristics, how efficiently some chemicals will penetrate the skin (See Table 2.2). If, for example, a pesticide is formulated in a vehicle based on xylenes a common practice for many emulsifiable concentrates of insecticides, then there is a near certainty that skin penetration by the pesticide will be accentuated. Because the xylene effect is largely, but not wholly, due to its effects on the cutaneous blood vessels[85] this marked effect on skin penetrability will not be apparent using isolated, *in vitro*, skin preparations.

4.4.3 Isolated respiratory tree

Some of the characteristics of inhalation exposure can be mimicked by the use of perfused respiratory trees extirpated from cadavers. As with many other isolated organ preparations the isolated system is effectively reduced to the function of its membrane properties and these are very different from the whole system functioning *in vivo*[511].

It is technically very difficult to devise isolated respiratory tree preparations that may be used to investigate uptake of gases, vapours, or aerosols and this is a severe limitation to the usefulness of these preparations for predictive acute toxicology[64,511].

Morphometric details of the respiratory tree have been studied by using casts and these provide some information on the likely distribution of particulates and aerosols entering the system[59]. Since uptake of particulates and aerosols is related more to their dynamic behaviour, rather than their static dimensions, this imposes a limitation on the usefulness of static anatomical models in inhalation toxicology[62].

It has been found that isolated organs can sometimes provide useful information about the uptake characteristics of toxicants and that they can be used to obtain important information on pharmacological action and toxico-kinetics with some classes of toxicants[673]. There are severe limitations associated with the use of isolated organs *in vitro* in bioavailability studies and in the main these methods are likely to be ancillary to, rather than replacements for, whole animal experiments carried out *in vivo*.

4.5   Invertebrates and Plants in Predictive Acute Toxicology

The majority of people concerned about the ethics of experimentation involving the use of living animals focus their attention on vertebrates. This is because vertebrate species are observed to be overtly sentient and many of the same people hold the opinion that invertebrates are incapable of suffering physical pain[294,448-454]. Some biologists consider that the cephalocordate animals possess nervous systems that are highly developed and that these animals, albeit inverte-brates, should be considered as sentient and that cephalocordate animals should be accorded the same humane principles as are considered acceptable for vertebrate species; however, cephalocordates are rarely used in predictive acute or sub-acute toxicology although they are sometimes used in investigative neurotoxicology.

Very large numbers of chemicals have been screened for possible insecticidal activity and the disparity of findings for any one chemical in different insect species does not give any reason to suppose that the correlation between insecticidal action and toxicity to vertebrates will be successful. Insecticidal activity is markedly influenced by bioavailability and as a possible model for vertebrate toxicity this bioavailability factor has to be taken into account. One approach has been the use of direct application of the chemicals to the insects by means of micro-applicators but available insecticidal data obtained in this way does not correlate well with known acute toxicology for the same chemicals in vertebrates. Although some metabolic pathways are similar in both insects and vertebrate animals, the overall physiological differences are so great that commonality is exceptional and this is a fundamental reason why it can never be assumed that a correlation exists between acute toxicity to vertebrates and invertebrates.

Because of the recognized importance of invertebrate species in the ecology of aquatic environmental systems there is an increasing awareness of the toxicology of environmental pollutants to these organisms. Thus there is a fund of data available from ecotoxicology studies that allows for review of the possible correlation between the toxicity of many chemicals to aquatic invertebrate species and also to vertebrate species[694]. No consistent correlation has been established between the toxicity of any chemical to aquatic invertebrate species and piscicidal properties, thus any correlation between toxicity to aquatic invertebrates and acute toxicity for terrestrial vertebrates would be unexpected.

In a detailed study of 75 chemicals using eight animal species, distributed between 2 phyla, 5 classes and 8 families, Kenega[512] concluded that it was possible to obtain useful predictive acute toxicity data for closely related species provided that they are within a class but not in different phyla. The same investigator[512] found no correlation between effects in terrestial and aquatic organisms. The usefulness of protozoa in some areas of toxicology has been established[513,514]. An example of the successful use of protozoa is attributable to Sovak and co-workers[515] who found an excellent correlation between the acute intravenous toxicities of several radiological contrast media and the corresponding LD_{50} [7 minutes] values to cultures of *Blepharisma americanum*; these investigators do not suggest that the use of this species has universal application as a model in acute toxicology and further they advise that caution is necessary in order to separate chemotoxicity from possible lethal effects on protozoa associated with viscosity and osmolarity.

There is substantial support for the use of microorganisms in predictive testing for carcinogenic and mutagenic potential but no correlation has been found between acute or sub-acute toxicity to vertebrates and microbiocidal properties. By selection of particular plants it is occasionally possible to develop models, generally based on plant biochemistry, that can be used to screen products for certain specific pharmacological activity[155]. The value of the whole plant, or selected processes associated with plant physiology, for the prediction of acute toxicity to vertebrate animals is extremely limited[516].

The poor correlation between responses observed among different vertebrate animals indicates that there can be little expectation of correlation between responses in organisms that are even more diverse in their whole physiology and biochemistry. This conclusion is supported by the extensive research into micro-biocides and pesticides which capitalizes on these fundamental differences.

4.6 Mathematical Models and Structure Action Relationships

With the development of computer technology and the great advances being made in the measurement of molecular characteristics there has been a realiza-tion of the potential for *in vitro* prediction of chemico–biological interactions[517-525]. Knowledge that physico–chemical properties are linked to biological reactivity is not new and the original idea is generally attributed[525] to two nineteenth Century scientists, Crum-Brown and Frazer, who were investigating the pharmacological activities of some alkaloids; their idea has subsequently been adapted and developed by many other investigators[527,528].

One of the first substantiated correlations between a physico–chemical characteristic and pharmacological, or toxicological, action was the fact that the lipid–water partition coefficients of some chemicals could be correlated with narcotic properties; the original observation is attributable to two independent investigators, Meyer who published his findings in 1899 and Overton who published in 1901, both of these scientists are acknowledged by the general title for the phenomenon known as the Overton–Meyer Hypothesis[529]. Since the origin of the Overton–Meyer Hypothesis there have been numerous other applications of lipid–water partition coefficients in the explanation of various toxicokinetic effects[530,531]. In terms of uptake of toxicants through the skin[239,532,641] and within the alimentary tract[533] the lipid–water partition coefficient is considered to be a particularly relevant characteristic of the product[618].

Bioaccumulation characteristics are often associated with acute and sub-acute toxic effects and the lipid–water partition coefficients of products are frequently found to be related to their ability to accumulate in the biosphere[534,535]. Although relationships between lipid–water partition coefficients, bioaccumulation and biological activity are convenient, because of the ease with which partition coefficients can be determined, caution in their application is necessary because the mathematical form of the correlation is a parabolic function rather than a linear relationship[534–538].

Although lipid–water partition coefficients are determinable it is more usual to use *n*-octanol, or more rarely *n*-heptanol, rather than lipids that are variable in composition. The accepted correlation between *n*-octanol/water, or *n*-heptanol/water, partition and lipid/water partition provides a convenient practical approach to one of the very important toxicokinetic principles[535–538].

Linear–free energy is a molecular characteristics that received early attention in relation to biological effects[526,539]. This has been followed by investigation of many other physical and chemical variables for an enormous variety of molecules and biological interactions [479,520–522,540–552]. The studies of structure action relationships (SAR) have developed to the stage of being a valuable predictive tool in many parmacological and toxicological research programmes[518,553–556]. The development of statistical methods[557] and computerised techniques[558,559] has made the handling of the large amount of complex physico–chemical data that is inevitably associated with SAR, more managable and many quantitative structure action relationships (QSAR) are now readily assessed.

Investigations involving QSAR are generally associated with the chemical biological interaction at the target rather than population effects. Physical and chemical properties, together with computerized mathematical techniques, are now widely used to predict toxicokinetic behaviour in general terms[560–564] but these methods still require extensive research and further development before they will significantly diminish the need for *in vivo* studies[564,565]. In a detailed study of QSAR data for 129 chemically related trifluoromethyl-benzimidazoles, Adamson and co-workers[566] concluded that the LD_{50} value is not a suitable end-point for correlative use in this type of investigation; if this conclusion is upheld for a series of chemicals with such common characteristics as these trifluoromethyl-benzimidazoles there can be little confidence in the QSAR approach for predicting LD_{50} values with chemicals that are dissimilar to each other.

A computerized QSAR system for predicting LD_{50} values has been developed[517,567] but some doubts about the applicability of this system have been published[518,568]. It has been claimed for this system that it is capable of predicting LD_{50} values, as determined in the laboratory rat, with a high level of success. As the QSAR data base increases the importance of this *in vitro* method, as a replacement for the conventional rodent LD_{50} test, will also increase and the findings obtained will become more credible. Acute toxicity measured in terms of LD_{50} values obtained using laboratory rodents is not in itself free from scientific criticism and this must be taken into account when assessing the shortcomings of QSAR approaches to assessment, especially when the rodent LD_{50} values are used as the correlate for the *in vitro* findings (see Section 3.4).

4.7 Reduction in Quantity of Animals used by Experimental Design

It is generally accepted that there is a need for some means of predicting acute toxic potential but most investigators would welcome methodology that did not involve the use of sentient living animals. In the current state of knowledge it is clear that no complete replacement of living animals by *in vitro* technology is yet available. The importance of refinement of methodology as means of diminishing need for the use of living animals for this aspect of toxicology is accentuated.

The importance of both qualitative and quantitative aspects of acute toxicology have been discussed and the underlying principles associated with the LD_{50} assessment have been explained (Chapter 3). The LD_{50} test has become firmly entrenched in the requirements for various health and safety regulations because it is technically easy to provide a convenient index of acute toxicity for a modest financial cost. Now the LD_{50} test has become a *bête noire* to those people with an antipathy to experimentation involving the use of sentient animals and also to many toxicologists[569-572] and the emphasis is changing from quantitative indices, based on large populations, to more detailed studies requiring less animals. In order to comply with the basic desire for quantification in acute toxicology, whether the desire is to create statistical respectability or, perhaps more justifiably, in order to have the convenience of a numeric index of acute toxicity for classification purposes, improving experimental design is receiving a lot more attention[163,221,230,569-573].

The method of 'moving averages' or variations on the 'up-and-down' ('pyramid') method can be used to reduce the number of animals required in acute toxicity testing[574,660,661]. Reducing the number of animals used in the assessment of median lethal doses will inevitably widen the confidence limits that have to be applied to the estimate[170,203,221,575,642] and information on the slope of the dose–response may be less reliable[170,203,230]; investigators have to decide on the level of precision that is necessary for a particular acute toxicity test whilst accepting that results from predictive acute toxicology are never accurate[618,622]. It is important to remember that the slope of the exposure response relationship may be more important than the LD_{50} value in isolation[640] and that this information may not be apparent in abbreviated LD_{50} tests.

Guidelines for the actual numbers of animals required to investigate the sub-acute toxicology of any product tend to be, of necessity, rather speculative. The development of any sub-acute investigative study requires careful planning with a thorough definition of the objectives. Some studies will involve comparisons of biological variables (e.g. body and organ weights; changes in the physiological chemistry; haematological data, etc.) and it becomes essential that the population of animals used is adequate for statistically meaningful comparisons to be made[210-214]. If the sub-acute investigation is only required to be a fairly crude guide as to whether cumulative toxicity occurs, as manifested by overt signs of intoxication, then small numbers of animals may be all that are required to provide adequate information. Whatever the objectives, sub-acute toxicity testing must be carried out using the minimum numbers of animals compatible with obtaining meaningful results.

5

The Intrinsic Importance of Predictive Acute and Sub-acute Toxicity Testing

It is not possible to quantify, other than very approximately, the number of chemicals that exist. In 1982, in a publication orginating from the World Health Organization, it was estimated that there were about four million known chemicals and that the number increases at the rate of about one thousand each year[604]. If this figure is accepted as being a reasonable estimate, then the enormous scale of possibilities associated with acute and sub-acute toxicology becomes immediately apparent. Each individual chemical possesses an intrinsic toxicity potential that will vary with route of exposure, target species, etc; some are extremely toxic whereas others are less toxic.

The potential hazards associated with exposures to more than one chemical makes the spectrum of toxic possibilities almost infinite because acute and sub-acute intoxications are not restricted to individual chemicals. Superimposed on this are the influences of numerous extraneous factors such as ambient conditions and the health status of the target animals.

Historically predictive toxicology has developed as an amalgamation of qualitative observations, usually associated with the clinical sciences, coupled with a desire for the quasi-respectability of quantification common to the physical sciences. It is a matter for conjecture as to whether predictive acute and sub-acute toxicology have benefited from, or been retarded by, the pragmatism that has characterized much of toxicology. (Historically many toxicologists have been prepared to accept the practicable rather than the ideal courses of action; many toxicologists argue that, in the main, the results have justified the means).

Confused thinking is frequently manifested by the misguided opinion that LD_{50} values possess intrinsic properties making them more than convenient indices of acute toxicity; there are now numerous publications seeking to set the record straight[154,155,163,449,455,570,571,574,605]. It would be quite wrong to conclude that LD_{50} values have no honourable purpose, rather it is that too many people have abused the validity of LD_{50} values by failing to apply good scientific judgement in their usage[574]. Used properly, the LD_{50} value has legitimate applications but indiscriminate use must be constrained[155].

For many purposes it is sufficient to have clear descriptive definitions of the acute toxicology of products without the need for numeric indices, in other words, the application of descriptive criteria such as 'extremely toxic' to 'almost non-toxic'. Under these circumstances precise quantification is unnecessary and an approximate idea of the toxic exposure level is all that is required[163]. This amount of quantification can be achieved by tests involving the use of small numbers of experimental animals[569-572,642] and, hopefully will eventually be replaced by methodology that does not necessitate the use of sentient animals at all[155]. Toxicologists and any other people associated with the problems of acute intoxication, must always make full use of the accumulated experience with products and not perpetuate testing, in the format of the LD_{50} test, without due cause. As long ago as 1957, the Secretary-General of the Universities Federation for Animal Welfare (UFAW)*, wrote [613], 'one cannot help wondering how far the extensive use of the 50% survival test is a hangover due to habit and custom and whether suitable continuous variates have been sought as diligently as could be desired'. Now, more than a quarter of a century later, that same line of thought has been adopted by many other people.

The possibility that misleading results will arise from using too few animals in predictive testing is real but the justification for using large populations for testing has also been challenged by many experienced toxicologists[163,570,571].

There are several published accounts of attempts at validation of the reproducibility of acute toxicity tests carried out within individual laboratories[576-578] and also the findings of collaborative investigations carried out involving several laboratories[577-581]. In addition it is common knowledge that there have been many unpublished investigations that have been carried out within laboratories to check reproducibility of data. The overall conclusion from these studies is that there is a remarkable lack of reproducibility of quantitative findings, both within and between laboratories, and that this is coupled with a disturbing degree of poor reporting of relevant observations by some investigators.

The median lethal dose, generally expressed as the LD_{50} value, does serve as a useful index of acute toxicity for classification of products for regulatory purposes but the caveats that must be attached to the logical use of LD_{50} data are frequently omitted from classification systems. The World Health Organization classification of pesticides[614] has merit in this respect as it classifies all pesticides into named classes ranging from 'extremely hazardous' to 'unlikely to present any acute hazard in normal use', this classification is based mainly on LD_{50} data but with cognizance of the overriding importance of taking into account relevant ancillary information. The fundamental principle of the World Health Organization classification[614] is acute risk to human health; thus if there is information to suggest that the LD_{50} value for a pesticide, or any of its formulations might be misleading in respect of human health then the LD_{50} values can be disregarded as the index of acute toxicity. Examples of the application of this caveat are found among pesticides that cause delayed neuro-pathies although some of these neurotoxic compounds have favourable LD_{50} values.

In addition to the World Health Organization classification of pesticides[614] there are numerous other classifications of products based on LD_{50} values[588]. It would not be particularly helpful to examine each of these classifications in detail here, however, it is pertinent to question the logistics underlying choice

*Universities Federation for Animal Welfare (UFAW), 8, Hamilton Close, Potters Bar, Herts. EN6 3QD, England.

of test species and also the required routes of exposure demanded for some classifications.

Most regulatory acute toxicity classifications address the relationship between acute toxicity assessed in animals and the likely effects on human health but not all acute toxicity testing is carried out for the purpose of predicting effects in man. Whenever extrapolation of findings from one species to another species is necessitated there can be major differences in response. This is exemplified by the large differences in sensitivity to acute intoxication found for different rodent species exposed to rodenticides. At first sight it seems more plausible to extrapolate data from one rodent species to another rodent species than from laboratory rats to man and yet the latter is often done uncritically[312]. Species variation is not limited to terrestial vertebrates and similar large differences are found in the relative sensitivities of different fish species and in different species of birds.

Species differences in sensitivity to intoxication highlight the need for the logical use of multi-species studies, with concomitant detailed investigation of the responses, rather than statistically based experiments using numerous animals of one species only[292,293]. Until such time as as replacement for sentient animals can be found it will be necessary to concentrate on reduction of the numbers of animals used by refinement of the investigative methods[638]. Well designed and competently performed investigations based on multiple species rather than large populations of one species fits the criteria of the reduction and refinement objectives but clearly is not a replacement of animals in investigative toxicology.

The idea of the '3R's' (reduction, refinement and replacement) in relation to the whole field of animal experimentation is receiving support, both in practice and in principle, from various responsible organizations and this support is apparent in relation to the LD_{50} test. The international pharmaceutical industry has become outspoken in this subject and in the USA the Pharmaceutical Manufacturing Association* has made public their opinion that:

(i) 'Seen as part of a battery of studies, the classical LD_{50} test which utilizes many animals to determine an LD_{50} value with mathematical precision lacks justification. Regulatory requirements should accommodate this position.'

(ii) 'While cautioning that the use of animals in acute safety studies remain essential the Pharmaceutical Manufacturers Association urges members to obtain a maximum amount of scientific information from the use of minimum numbers of animals.'

This clear statement[582] is very much in accord with the spirit of the 'Report on the LD_{50} Test' that was prepared in the UK, in 1970 and presented to the Secretary of State by the Advisory Committee on the Administration of the Cruelty to Animals Act, 1876.** It is also entirely compatible with current thinking in Europe[455,569–572,605–607].

*Pharmaceutical Manufacturers Association, 1100 Fifteenth Street, N.W., Washington DC 20005, USA.
**In the UK any acute or sub-acute toxicity investigations involving the use of vertebrate animals were controlled by the provisions of the Cruelty to Animals Act, 1876. With effect from 1 January 1987 new legislation came into force as the Animals (Scientific Procedures) Act, 1986.

Although information from acute and sub-acute toxicity testing are used for various forms of risk–benefit analysis it is not always possible to cover the conditions of all risk situations and a review of the incidence of cases of intoxication does not engender confidence that all of the effort that has been dedicated to predictive testing has been justified. There is no way of assessing whether the situation would have been worse if there had been no predictive testing but clearly it could not be better. Pesticides are extensively tested for their acute toxicity potential and are subject to World Health Organization and other classification systems[614,615]. In the UK, and many other Western Countries, the safety record for pesticides, in terms of acute intoxication of humans, is excellent if deliberate self-destruction (i.e. suicide and attempted suicide) is omitted from the recorded incidence[583,584]. The influence of socio-economic factors on the overall incidence of human intoxication is important and this is immediately apparent with the distribution of reported cases of acute pesticide intoxication throughout the USA. Once the Third World is included in the review the incidence of acute intoxication by pesticides becomes unacceptably large; but reliable data for Third World countries are difficult to establish because of inadequate surveillance and available information is sometimes challenged. An estimate of the incidence of cases of acute intoxications attributable to pesticides in the Third World was published in 1982[585] and, at that time, the lowest estimate was 187 000 people affected including 5000 deaths and the figures may be substantially bigger. More recently the World Health Organization[614] has put these figures at about 500 000 cases of pesticide poisoning resulting in 5000 deaths each year and it is accepted by the World Health Organization that this is probably an underestimate. It was found that in 1987, Guyana, actually imported thallium sulphate, (*note*: importation estimated to be 5000 kg of this chemical per year), to kill rats in sugar plantations. Thallium salts have a reputation as toxicants[646] and their use as rodenticides is totally against World Health Organization recommendations. Many deaths have occurred among the people of Guyana as a direct result of thallium poisoning and it is known that a large part of the Guyanese population are carrying potentially toxic body burdens of thallium[662]. No amount of predictive toxicology seems able to prevent human folly.

Analyses of risk–benefit relationships are difficult even for those products that may appear to have well defined use patterns[586]. In reality risk–benefit equations are generally too simplistic and some of the necessary objectivity required for this type of analysis may be lost when commercial expediency is allowed to influence the process. There are many questions that can be posed in the assessment of risk–benefit and yet inevitably the answers to those questions will be variable and subjective[13]. For example, how are the merits of a drug that is beneficial to some severely ill patients ranked when the same product is known to produce manifestations of acute intoxication, possibly lethal, in a proportion of those exposed[695]? Similarly, how can the life-saving properties of pesticides that are available to eradicate the vectors of debilitating, often fatal diseases, or pesticides that make it possible to grow edible crops in those parts of the World in which malnutrition and starvation are endemic, be off-set against the possibility of an incidence of intoxication[683]? Clearly there are no simple answers to questions such as these and they are doomed to remain as emotive socio-political debating points. The contribution of toxicology to risk–benefit analysis is greatly weakened if predictions are not based on scientifically credible investigations.

Sometimes information on the toxic potential of a product is confounded by events. It is possible to have an extensive knowledge of the toxicology of a product, including data from exposed humans and from laboratory tests, and yet have the validity of the information set aside because of impurities that may have arisen during the manufacturing process or during storage[587]. To illustrate this point it is only necessary to consider the *cause célèbre* of recent years when it was found that the herbicide 2,4,5-T, which has a very favourable acute toxicity rating, could be contaminated during production by the extremely toxic compound 2,3,7,8-tetrachlorodibenzo-*p*-dioxin[588,589,644]. Similarly, malathion is an insecticide with a favourable acute toxicity rating[614], and a long history of safety in use, but if malathion is stored at elevated temperatures formation of highly toxic by-products occurs. Large quantities of malathion are used in tropical countries and the expected safety margin may be reduced unless the product is carefully stored[590,591]. It is possible for impurities and contaminants to reduce the acute toxicity potential of a product but this effect is generally less obvious[590]. Sometimes, in an attempt to reduce the risk of intoxication, various additives are included in formulations, in other words, the inclusion of intensely bitter tasting additives (e.g. denatonium benzoate) or additives that impart an extremely unpleasant odour (e.g. some thio-compounds) but this approach to safety must not be confused with the intrinsic toxicological interactions described elsewhere (see Section 3.3.). A further approach to the reduction of acute risk is the inclusion of emetics (e.g. ipecacuanha) in formulations but this is not without its own additional hazard (i.e. emesis can lead to aspiration) and the use of ipecacuanha in the treatment of acute intoxication has been criticized[643].

The acute toxicity potentials of products may be important in disaster situations and, in turn, the toxic potential may be influenced by the conditions of the disaster. Interactions often occur during fires and explosions both of which can cause the spread of chemicals and may also cause different toxicants to be formed, as a result of pyrolysis, and released into the environment[588,592-594,608]. Perversely fire extinguishers and fire retardants have been implicated as toxicants[595] and it is often found that people are affected, sometimes killed, as a result of acute intoxication by toxic vapours given off during conflagrations; this has considerable impact on the design and fabrication requirements for buildings, furnishings and fittings and the Fire and Rescue Services often find that inadequate attention has been given to these aspects of safety.

There is a fairly common misconception that man alone is responsible for generating toxic chemicals. Some of the most toxic chemicals are formed in nature by microorganisms[596,609], plants[597,598] and animals[599-602]. Both invertebrates and vertebrates are capable of producing extremely toxic chemicals and these are generally called 'toxins' to distinguish them from synthetic toxicants. Many, but not all, toxins originating from animals and microorganisms are proteins[599-601].

An idea of the extremely toxic nature of some toxins can be gained by reference to the acute toxicity of the proteins that comprise the exotoxin produced by the microorganism *Clostridium botulinum*; this toxin is lethal to mice, by the intraperitoneal route, at approximately 1.5×10^{-6} mg kg^{-1}. Botulism, which is the name given to intoxication by the exotoxin from *Clostridium botulinum*, has been the cause of many human deaths. Although the importance of toxicokinetic studies in relation to acute toxicology is recognized[603] and these studies form an integral part of investigations into acute intoxication it is technically difficult to investigate the toxicokinetics of proteins that are intensely toxic at such physiological dilution levels[16].

Predictive acute toxicity testing has been the subject of justifiably severe criticism, for too often investigators have been satisfied with testing procedures that are inadequate[685]. There has been excessive interest in statistical nicety rather than with the establishment of realistic objectives[569-574,615,616]. Legislative requirements, rather than ethical and moral implications of experimentation, have been the overriding influences for some investigators and the search for alternatives to the use of sentient animals in acute toxicology has been slow. The fact that it is possible to reduce the numbers of animals used in acute and sub-acute toxicology by refining experimental procedures is now recognized[638] and the fact that refined testing procedures might lead to more meaningful results is a worthwhile bonus[685]. In comparison with the financial costs associated with the discovery and development of most new products, the economies that can be made in predictive acute and sub-acute toxicity testing do not offer significant savings, thus some cynics attribute slow progress in the search for alternatives to lack of financial incentive but this is an over simplistic explanation.

In order to minimize the necessity for replication of testing it is necessary for all valid acute toxicity tests to be documented and the findings from these tests made available through data retrieval systems. In addition to the legitimate confidentiality attributable to some information there are severe logistic problems associated with data banking in toxicology. The practical problems associated with adequately cataloguing detailed acute toxicity data has reinforced the popularity of LD_{50} values as convenient indices of acute toxic potential; LD_{50} values have the merit of easy retrieval and ready reference and, regrettably, the limited nature of the information is frequently overlooked.

Any credible data banking system must have the capability of having the quality of data input monitored. No currently available system has the ability to censor its own input, thus the user of the system has to choose whether to accept data at face value or, alternatively, checking on the information by replication of the testing. Ideally the findings from all acute toxicity testing would be published as detailed contributions to the scientific literature, that way all of the information would be readily available and data would be professionally reviewed before publication; unfortunately the practicability of this approach makes it impossible to achieve without a considerable change in attitudes and a very large increase in the resources associated with publications.

This monograph has been produced in order to provide an insight into the underlying principles of predictive acute and sub-acute toxicology. The various strengths and weaknesses of available and established methodology have been reviewed and hopefully this may stimulate a more critical approach to predictive acute and sub-acute toxicology. Although most predictive toxicology has developed as a pragmatic branch of science there is an increasing awareness that the long established methodology used in acute and sub-acute toxicity testing, with its inclination towards quantification, needs constructive rethinking and that the use of sentient animals for this purpose should only be undertaken when no realistic alternative is available. However, just as every investigator must apply stringent ethical principles to any decision to carry out any investigation involving the use of sentient animals it is also necessary to be aware of the moral and legal implications governing the use of humans for investigative purposes[150,610-612] and also to take cognizance of the possible consequences of not having adequate information about the toxic potential of any product.

Predictably the attitude of the community at large to matters of acute toxicology is illogical but it is the ambivalence exhibited by professional toxicologists that is most surprising.

Too often it needs a disaster, or at least a near disaster, to trigger research in acute toxicology. Such disasters as the contaminated edible oil syndrome in Spain or the Bhopal pesticide manufacturing plant incident serve to highlight the fact that accumulated wisdom is either inadequate or not applied in situations where it matters. What constitutes a disaster, and hence facilitates the perceived need for research in acute toxicology, is difficult to define. The events at Seveso that led to the release of toxic polychlorinated chemicals into the environment is rated by most people as a 'disaster' and yet it is probable that no deaths occurred as a direct result of acute intoxication of humans[644]. A prodigeous amount of research into the acute toxicology of these polychlorinated chemicals has followed the Seveso incident[644]. Conversely, in England and Wales alone (UK Government figures) the death toll in one typical year (1983) due to analgesics, including aspirin, was 116 people. In a period of two decades (1958 to 1977) the deaths of 598 children in England, Scotland and Wales alone were registered as being due to poisoning[645]. The research response hardly matches that which would be anticipated if the same number died in a 'disaster'.

It is time that professional ambivalence should be removed and the future needs of toxicology in respect of acute and sub-acute exposures appraised and a more meaningful approach implemented.

References

1. Rymer, M.M. and Fishman, R.A., Protective adaptation of brain to water intoxication, *Neurology*, 1972, **22**, 397.
2. Boyd, E.M. and Godi, I., Acute oral toxicity of distilled water in albino rats, *Ind. Med. Surg.*, 1967, **36**, 609.
3. Richardson, J.A. and Pratt-Thomas, H.E., Toxic effects of varying doses of kerosene administered by different routes, *Am. J. Med. Sci.*, 1951, **221**, 531.
4. Narasimhan, M.J., Jr., and Ganla, V.G., Experimental studies on kerosene poisoning, *Acta Pharmacol. Toxicol.*, 1967, **25**, 214.
5. Grover, J., Acute poisoning, *Armed Forces Med. J. (India)*, 1971, **27**, 358.
6. Brown, V.K.H., Box, V.L. and Simpson, B.J., Decontamination procedures for skin exposed to phenolic substances, *Arch. Environ. Hlth.*, 1975, **30**, 1.
7. Beaven, M.A., Anaphylactoid reactions to anaesthetic drugs, *Anaesthesiology*, 1981, **5**, 3.
8. Mantz, J.M., Pauli, G., Meyer, P., Tempe, J.D., Jaeger, A., Kopferschmidt, J., Sasuder, J.J., Flesch, J.J. and Bennett, A., Le choc anaphylactique: resultats d'une enquete nationale portant sur 1047 cas, *Rev. Med. Intern.*, 1982, **3**, 331.
9. Silverglade, A., Cardiac toxicity of aerosol propellants, *J. Am. Med. Assoc.*, 1972, **222**, 827.
10. Clark, D.G. and Tinston, D.J., Acute inhalation toxicity of some halogenated and non-halogenated hydrocarbons, *Human Toxicology*, 1982, **1**, 239.
11. *Principles for Evaluating Chemicals in the Environment.* A report of the Committee for the Working Conference on Principles of Protocols for Evaluating Chemicals in the Environment. *National Academy of Sciences, Washington DC*, 1975.
12. Hagan, E.C., Acute toxicity, in *Appraisal of the Safety of Chemicals in Foods, Drugs and Cosmetics*, Association of Food and Drug Officials of the United States, 1959.
13. Marshall, V., Hazard-risk-which?, *Health and Safety at Work*, 1981, **3**, 52.
14. Vale, J.A. and Meredith, T.J., Poisons information services, in *Poisoning: Diagnosis and Treatment*, Eds., Vale, J.A. and Meredith, T.J., Update Books, London, Dordrecht and Boston., 1983, 5.
15. Gresham, G.A. and Mashru, M.K.S., Fatal poisoning with sodium chloride, *Forensic Sci. Int.*, 1982, **20**, 87.
16. Freyvogel, T.A. and Perret, B.A., Notes on toxinology, *Experientia*, 1972, **29**, 1317.
17. van Rossum, J.M. and Burgers, J.P.T., Quantitative relationship between dynamics and kinetics of drugs: A systems dynamics approach, *Drug Metabolism Revs.*, 1984, **15**, 365.
18. van Rossum, J.M., van Lingen, G. and Burgens, J.B.P., Dose-dependent pharmacokinetics, *Pharm. Ther.*, 1983, 211, 77.

19. Tallarida, R.J., Receptor theories and quantitative effect versus dose–concentration relationship *Drug Metabolism Revs.*, 1984, **15**, 345.

20. Prestcott, L.F., Paracetamol overdosage: Pharmacological considerations and clinical management, *Drugs*, 1983, **25**, 290.

21. Moffat, A.C., Absorption of drugs through the oral mucosa, in *Absorption Phenomena*, Eds., Rabinowitz, J. and Myerson, R., Wiley-International, 1971, 1.

22. Lien, E., Koda, R.T. and Tong, G.L., Buccal and percutaneous absorptions, *Drug Intel. Clin. Pharm.*, 1971, **5**, 38.

23. Beckett, A.H. and Hoosie, R.D., Buccal absorption of drugs, in *Concepts in Biochemical Pharmacology*, Eds., Brodie, B.B. and Gillette, J.R., Handbook of Experimental Pharmacology, Eds., Eichler, B., Farah, A., Herken, H. and Welch, A.D., Springer-Verlag, 1971, 25.

24 Ho, N.F.H., and Higuchi, W.I., Quantitative interpretation of *in vivo* buccal absorption of *n*-alkanoic acids by the physical model approach, *J. Pharm. Sci.*, 1971, **60**, 537.

25. Dollery, C.T. and Davies, D.S., Routes of administration and drug response, in *Concept in Biochemical Pharmacology*, Pt. 3, Eds., Gillette, J.R. and Mitchell, J.R., Springer-Verlag, 1975.

26. Agular, A.J., Physical properties and pharmaceutical manipulations influencing drug absorption, in *Pharmacology of intestinal absorption: Gastro-intestinal absorption of Drugs*, 1, Eds., Forth, W. and Rummel, W., Pergamon Press, 1975, 335.

27. Schanker, L.S., On the mechanism of absorption of drugs from the gastro-intestinal tract, *J. Med. Pharm. Chem.*, 1960, **2**, 343.

28. Kurz, H., Principles of drug absorption, in *Pharmacology of intestinal absorption: Gastro-intestinal absorption of Drugs*, 1, Eds., Forth, W. and Rummel, W., Pergamon Press, 1975, 245.

29. Parsons, D.S., Physiological and biochemical implications of intestinal absorption, in *Pharmacology of intestinal absorption: Gastro-intestinal absorption of Drugs*, 1, Eds., Forth, W. and Rummel, W., Pergamon Press, 1975, 71.

30. Florence, A.T., Design of medicines for oral administration: I Physical chemistry of drugs in relation to drug absorption, *Pharm. J.*, 1974, **213**, 264.

31. Smith, H.W., Observations on the flora of the alimentary tract of animals and factors affecting its composition, *J. Pathol. Bacteriol.*, 1965, **89**, 95.

32. Schanker, L.S., Shore, P.A., Brodie, B.B. and Hogben, C.A.M., Absorption of drugs from the stomach: I The rat, *J. Pharmacol. exptl. Ther.*, 1957, **120**, 528.

33. Hogben, C.A.M., Schanker, L.S., Tocco, D.J. and Brodie, B.B., Absorption of drugs from the stomach: II The human, *J. Pharmacol. exptl. Ther.*, 1957, **120**, 540.

34. Welling, P.G., Influence of food and diet on gastro-intestinal drug absorption: A review, *J. Pharmacokin. Biopharm.*, 1977, **5**, 291.

35. Watanabe, J., Okabe, H., Ichihashi, T., Mizojiri, K., Yamada, H. and Yamamoto, R., Gastric emptying rate constants after oral administration of drug solution to mice, rats and rabbits, *Chem. Pharm. Bull.*, 1977, **25**, 2147.

36. Melander, A., Influence of food on the bioavailability of drugs, *Clin. Pharmacokin.*, 1978, **3**, 337.

37. Tohyama, K., Horiguchi, Y. and Takeda, Y., Inhibition of gastric emptying by chloroform and its relation to strain differences in acute toxicity of chloroform in mice, *Tox. Letters*, 1983, **18**, 7.

38. Achord, J.L., Acute effects of fasting on gastro-intestinal structure and functioning, *Med. Times*, 1967, **95**, 441.
39. Dowling, R.H., Compensating changes in intestinal absorption, *Brit. Med. Bull.*, 1967, **23**, 275.
40. Apostelou, A., Saidt, L. and Brown, W.R., Effect of overnight fasting of young rats on water consumption, body weight; blood sampling and blood composition, *Lab. Anim. Sci.*, 1976, **2**, 959.
41. Houston, J.B., Upshall, D.G. and Bridges, J.W., The re-evaluation of the importance of partition coefficients in the gastro-intestinal absorption of nutrients, *J. Pharmacol. exptl. Ther.*, 1974, **189**, 244.
42. Houston, J.B., Upshall, D.G. and Bridges, J.W., Further studies using carbamate esters as model compounds to investigate the role of lipophilicity in the gastro-intestinal absorption of foreign compounds, *J. Pharmacol. exptl. Ther.*, 1975, **195**, 67.
43. Lanman, R.C., Stremsterfer, C.E. and Schanker, L.S., Absorption of organic anions from the rat small intestine, *Xenobiotica*, 1971, **1**, 613.
44. Lecce, J.G., Absorption of macromolecules by mammalian intestinal epithelium, in *Intestinal Toxicology*, Ed., Schiller, C.M., Raven Press, 1984.
45. Kuksij, A., Intestinal digestion and absorption of fat-soluble environmental agents, in *Intestinal Toxicology*, Ed., Schiller, C.M., Raven Press, 1984.
46. Steenbock, H., Irwin, M.H., Weber, J. Templin. V.M., Pickering, M.A., Kemmerer, A.R. and Lease, E.J., Comparative rate of absorption of different fats, *J. Nutrition*, 1936, **12**, 103.
47. Dolvisio, J.T., Tan, G.H., Billups, N.F. and Diamond, L., Drug absorption: II Effect of fasting on intestinal drug absorption, *J. Pharm. Sci.*, 1969, **58**, 1200.
48. Diamond, L., Dolvisio, J.T. and Crouthamel, W.G., Physiological factors affecting drug absorption, *Europ. J. Pharmacol.*, 1970, **11**, 109.
49. Kitazawa, S. and Komuro, T., Effect of fasting on body fluids and intestinal drug absorption in rats, *Chem. Pharm. Bull.*, 1977, **25**, 327.
50. Kast, A. and Nishikawa, J., Effect of fasting on oral acute toxicity of drugs in rats and mice, *Lab. Animals*, 1981, **15**, 359.
51. Welling, P.G. and Tse, F.L.S., Food interactions affecting the absorption of anti-inflammatory agents, *Drug–Nutrient Interactions*, 1983, **2**, 153.
52. Hoensch, H.P. and Schwank, M., Intestinal absorption and metabolism of xenobiotics in humans, in *Intestinal Toxicology*, Ed., Schiller, C.M., Raven Press, 1984.
53. Johnson, H.D. and Voss, E., Toxicological studies of zinc phosphide, *J. Am. Pharm. Assoc.*, (Sci. Ed.), 1952, **41**, 468.
54. Riegelman, S. and Crowall, W.J., The kinetics of rectal absorption: I Preliminary investigations into the absorption rate process, *J. Amer. Pharm. Assoc., (Sci. Ed.)*, 1958, **47**, 115.
55. Riegelman, S. and Crowall, W.J., The kinetics of rectal absorption: II The absorption of animals, *J. Amer.Pharm. Assoc., (Sci. Ed.)*, 1958, **47**, 123.
56. De Boer, A.G. and Breimer, D.D., Rectal absorption: Portal or systemic, in *Drug Absorption*, Eds., Prescott, L.F. and Nimmo, W.S., MTP Press Ltd., Lancaster, 1979, 61.
57. Wilson, A.G.E., Toxicokinetics of uptake, accumulation and metabolism of chemicals by the lung, in *Mechanisms in Respiratory Toxicology*, Vol. 1, Eds., Witschi, H.R. and Nettlesheim, P., CRC Press Inc; Boca Raton, 1982, 161.
58. Alarie, Y., Toxicological evaluation of airborne chemical irritants and allergens using respiratory reflex reactions, in *Inhalation Toxicology and*

Technology, Ed., Leons, B.K.J., Ann Arbor Science Publishers Inc., Ann Arbor, 1981, 207.

59. Schlesinger, R.B., Particle deposition in model systems of human and experimental animal airways, in *Generation of Aerosols and facilities for Exposure Experiments*, Ed., Willeke, K., Ann Arbor Science Publishers Inc., Ann Arbor, 1980.

60. Halbert, M.K., Mazumder, M.K. and Bond, R.L., Respirable particulates in household aerosols, *Environ. Res.*, 1981, **26**, 105.

61. Vincent, J.H. and Armbruster, L., On the Quantitative definition of the inhalability of airborne dust, *Am. Occup. Hyg.*, 1981, **24**, 245.

62. Morrow, P.E., Evaluation of inhalation hazards based upon the respirable dust concept and the philosophy and application of selective sampling, *Am. Industr. Hyg. Assoc. J.*, 1964, **25**, 213.

63. Rackow, H., Absorption, distribution and excretion of gaseous anaesthetics, in *Concepts in Biochemical Pharmacology Part 1*, Eds., Brodie, B.B. and Gillette, J.R., Springer-Verlag, 1971, 67.

64. Stott, W.T. and McKenna, M.J., The comparative absorption and excretion of chemical vapours by the upper, lower and intact respiratory tracts of rats, *Fund. Appl. Toxicol.*, 1984, **4**, 594.

65. Enna, S.J. and Schanker, L.S., Absorption of saccharides and urea from the rat lung, *Amer. J. Physiol.*, 1972a, **222**, 409.

66. Enna, S.J. and Schanker, L.S., Absorption of drugs from the rat lung, *Amer. J. Physiol.*, 1972b, **223**, 1227.

67. Agarwal, J.K., Remiarz, R.J. and Nelson, P.A., An instrument for real time aerodynamic particle size analysis using laser velocimetry, in *Inhalation Toxicology and Technology*, Ed., Leons, B.J.K., Ann Arbor Science Publishers Inc., Ann Arbor, 1981, 177.

68. Raabe, O.G., Generation and characterization of aerosols, in *Inhalation Carcinogenesis*, Ed., Hanna, M.G., Jr., Nettesheim, P. and Gilbert, J.R., US Atomic Energy Commission (Div. of Technical Information), Springfield, 1970.

69. Raabe, O.G., Deposition and clearance of inhaled aerosols, in *Mechanism in Respiratory Toxicology*, 1, Eds., Witschi, H. and Nettesheim, P., CRC Press Inc., Boca Raton, 1982, 27.

70. Morrison, P.E., Some physical and physiological factors controlling the fate of inhaled substances, *Health Physics*, 1960, **2**, 366.

71. Beeckmans, J.M., The deposition of aerosols in the respiratory tract: I Mathematical analysis and comparison with experimental data, *Canad. J. Physiol. Pharmacol.*, 1965, **43**, 157.

72. Yeh, H–C., Phalen, R.F. and Raabe, O.G., Factors influencing the deposition of inhaled particles, *Environ. Hlth. Perspect.*, 1976, **15**, 147.

73. Lippman, M. and Albert, R.E., The effect of particle size on the regional deposition of inhaled aerosols in the human respiratory tract, *Am. Industr. Hyg. Assoc. J.*, 1969, **30**, 257.

74. Thomas, R.G., Estimation of particle size distribution parameters in animal lungs, *Aerosol Sci.*, 1971, **2** 393.

75. Sanockij, I.V., Methods for determining toxicity and hazards of chemicals, quoted in *Principles and Methods for Evaluating the Toxicity of Chemicals*, Part I, (Environmental Health Criteria 6), World Health Organisation, Geneva, 1978.

76. Yeh, H–C and Schum, G.M., Models of human lung airways and their application to inhaled particle deposition, *Bull. Math. Biol.*, 1980, **42**, 461.

77. Rothman, S., *Physiology and Biochemistry of the skin*, University of Chicago Press, Chicago, 1954.

78. Mier, P.D. and Cotton, D.W.K., *The Molecular Biology of Skin*, Blackwell Scientific Publications, 1971.

79. Maibach, H.I., Feedmann, R.J., Milby, T. and Serat, W.F., Regional variation in percutaneous penetration in man, *Arch. Environ. Hlth.*, 1971, **23**, 208.

80. Webster, R.C. and Noonan, P.K., Relevance of animal models for percutaneous absorption, *Int. J. Pharmaceutics*, 1980, **7**, 99.

81. Reifenrath, W.G., Chellguist, E.M., Shipwash, E.A. and Jederberg, W.W., Evaluation of animal models for predicting skin penetration in man, *Fund. Appl. Toxicol.*, 1984, **4**, S224.

82. Katz, M. and Poulsen, B.J., Absorption of drugs through the skin, in *Concepts in Biochemical Pharmacology, Pt. 1*, Eds., Brodie, B.B. and Gillette, J.R., Handbook of Experimental Pharmacology XXXVIII/1, Eds., Eichler, O., Farah, A., Herken, H. and Welch, A.D., Springer-Verlag, 1971.

83. Grasso, P., Some aspects of the role of skin appendages in percutaneous absorption, *J. Soc. Cosmet. Chem.*, 1971, **22**, 523.

84. Albery, W.J., Guy, R.K. and Hadgraft, J., Percutaneous absorption: Transport in the dermis, *Int. J. Pharmaceutics*, 1983, **15**, 125.

85. Brown, V.K. and Box, V.L., Influence of some solvents on the vascularity of skin in relation to effects on systemic intoxication by solutes. Proceedings of 13th Meeting of the European Society for the Study of Drug Toxicity – Berlin (Excerpta Medica International Congress Series No. 254), 1971.

86. Dyer, A., Hayes, G.G., Wilson, J.G. and Catterall, R., Diffusion through skin and model systems, *Int. J. Cosmet. Sci.*, 1979, **1**, 91.

87. Barry, B.W., *Dermatological Formulations Percutaneous Absorption*, Marcel Dekker Inc., New York and Basel, 1983.

88. Hawkins, G.S. Jr., and Reifenrath, W.G., Development of an *in vitro* model for determining the fate of chemicals applied to the skin, *Fund. Appl. Toxicol.*, 1983, **4**, S133.

89. Buerger, A.A., A theory of integremental penetration, *J. Theor. Biol.*, 1967, **14**, 66.

90. Scheuplein, R.J. and Blank, I.H., Permeability of the skin, *Physiol. Rev.*, 1971, **51**, 302.

91. Faucher, J.A. and Goddard, E.F., Interaction of keratinous substrates with sodium lauryl sulphate: II Permeation through stratum corneum, *J. Soc. Cosmet. Chem.*, 1978, **29**, 339.

92. Draize, J.H., Nelson, A.A. and Calvery, H.O., The percutaneous absorption of DDT in laboratory animals, *J. Pharmacol. exptl. Ther.*, 1944, **82**, 159.

93. Noakes, D.N. and Sanderson, D.M., A method for determining the dermal toxicity of pesticides, *Br. J. industr. Med.*, 1969, **26**, 59.

94. Schanker, L.S., Physiological transport of drugs in, *Advances in Drug Research*, Vol. 1, Eds., Harper, N.J. and Simmonds, A.B., Academic Press, 1964.

95. Doane, M., Jensen, A. and Dohlman, C., Penetration routes for topically applied eye medications, *Am. J. Ophthalmol.*, 1978, **85**, 383.

96. Leopold, I.H. and Krishna, N., Local use of anticholinesterase agents in ocular therapy in, *Cholinesterase and Anticholinesterase Agents*, Sub. Ed., Koelle, G.B., *Handbuch der Experimentellen Pharmakologic XV*, Eds., Eichler, O. and Farah, A., Springer-Verlag, 1963, 1051.

97. Natoff, I.L., Influence of the route of administration on the toxicity of some cholinesterase inhibitors, *J. Pharm. Pharmac.*, 1967, **19**, 612.

98. Lukas, G., Brindle, S.D. and Greengard, P., The route of absorption of intra-peritonealy administered compounds, *J. Pharm. exptl. Ther.*, 1971, **178**, 562.

99. Kruger, S., Greve, D.W. and Schueler, F.W., The absorption of fluid from the peritoneal cavity, *Arch. Int. Pharmacodyn.*, 1962, **137**, 173.

100. Ballard, B.E. and Menczel, E., Subcutaneous absorption kinetics of benzyl alcohol, *J. Pharm. Sci.*, 1967, **56**, 1476.

101. Ballard, B.E., Biopharmaceutical considerations in subcutaneous and intramuscular drug administration, *J. Pharm. Sci.*, 1968, **57**, 357.

102. Koichiro, H., Teruhisa, I. and Hideo, Y., Studies on the absorption of practically water-insoluble drugs following injection. II: Intramuscular absorption from aqueous suspensions in rats, *Chem. Pharm. Bull.*, 1981, **29**, 817.

103. Koichiro, H., Teruhisa, I. and Hideo, Y., Studies on the absorption of practically water-insoluble drugs following injection. I: Intramuscular absorption from water immiscible oil solutions in rats, *Chem. Pharm. Bull.*, 1981, **29**, 519.

104. Koichiro, H., Teruhisa, I. and Hideo, Y., Studies on the absorption of practicaly water-insoluble drugs following injection. V: Subcutaneous absorption in rats from solutions in water immiscible oils, *J. Pharm. Sci.*, 1982, **71**, 495.

105. Koichiro, H. and Hideo, Y., Studies on the absorption of practically water-insoluble drugs following injection VI: Subcutaneous absorption from aqueous suspensions in rats, *J. Pharm. Sci.*, 1982, **71**, 500.

106. Koichiro, H. and Hideo, Y., Studies on the absorption of practically water-insoluble drugs following injection. VII: Plasma concentrations after different subcutaneous doses of drug in aqueous suspension in rats, *J. Pharm. Sci.*, 1983, **72**, 602.

107. Koichiro, H. and Hideo, Y., Studies on the absorption of practically water-insoluble drugs following injection. VIII: Comparison of the subcutaneous absorption rates from aqueous suspensions in the mouse, rat and rabbit, *J. Pharm. Sci.*, 1983, **72**, 608.

108. Freedman, A.M. and Himwich, H.E., DFP: Site of injection and variation in response, *Am. J. Physiol.*, 1949, **156**, 125.

109. Coleman, I.W. and Patton, G.E., A mouse restraint for intracerebral injection, *Canad. J. Physiol. Pharmacol.*, 1965, **43**, 173.

110. Rainsford, K.D., Toxicity in the brain of organophosphate insecticides: Comparison of the toxicity of metabolites with parent compounds using an intracerebral injection method, *Pestic. Biochem. Physiol.*, 1978, **8**, 302.

111. Rall, D.P., Drug entry into brain and cerebrospinal fluid in, *Concepts in Biochemical Pharmacology* Pt. 1, Eds., Brodie, B.B. and Gillette, J.R., Springer-Verlag, 1971.

112. Bates, I.P., The blood-brain-barrier and central nervous system drug penetration, *Pharm. J.*, 1984, **232**, 265.

113. Ferguson, H.C., Dilution of dose and acute oral toxicity, *Tox. Appl. Pharmacol.*, 1962, **4**, 759.

114. Crawford, D.L., Sinnhuber, R.O., Stout, F.M., Oldfield, J.E. and Kaufmes, J.K., Acute toxicity of malonaldehyde, *Tox. Appl. Pharmacol.*, 1965, **7**, 826.

115. Goodman, L.S. and Gilman, A., *The Pharmacological Basis of Therapeutics*, Macmillan, New York, 1970.

116. Borowitz, J.L., Moore, P.F., Yim, G.K.W. and Miya, T.S., Mechanism of enhanced drug effects produced by dilution of the oral dose, *Tox. Appl. Pharmacol.*, 1971, **19**, 164.

117. Nelson, N.S. and Hoar, R.M., A small animal balling gun for oral administration of experimental compound, *Lab. Anim. Care*, 1969, **19**, 871.

118. Shani, J., Givant, Y. and Sulman, F.G., A capsule-feeder for small laboratory animals, *Lab. Anim. Care*, 1970, **20**, 1154.

119. Stanislaus, F., Schneider, G.F. and Hofrichter, G., Zue technik der verabrei-

chung von Arzneistoffen in fasterform an der Ratte. (in German), *Drug Research*, 1979, **29**, 186.

120. Lax, E.R., Militzer, K. and Trauschel, A., A simple method for oral administration of drugs in solid form to fully conscious rats, *Lab. Anim.*, 1983, **17**, 50.

121. Wagner, J.G., Kinetics of pharmacological response: 1. Proposed relationships between response and drug concentration in the intact animal and man, *J. Theor. Biol.*, 1968, **20**, 173.

122. Laduron, P.M., Criteria for receptor sites in binding studies, *Biochem. Pharmacol.*, 1984, **33**, 833.

123. Molinengo, L. and Orsett, M., The principle of non-specificity and acute toxicity, *TIPS*, 1984, **5**, 185.

124. Häber, F., Zue geschichte des Gaskrierges in, *Funf Vortrage aud den Jahren 1920-1923*, Julius Springer, Berlin, 1924.

125. MacFarland, H.N., Inhalation toxicology, *J.A.O.A.C.*, 1975, **58**, 689.

126. Hilado, C.J. and Huttlinger, P.A., Comparison of time to death, survival time and LT_{50}, *J. Combust. Tox.*, 1981, **8**, 33.

127. Uehleke, H., Drug absorption and toxicity in, *Drug Absorption*, Eds., Prescott, L.F. and Nimmo, W.S., MTP Press Ltd., Lancaster, 1979, 123.

128. Stavchansky, S., Martin, A. and Loper, A., Solvent system effects on drug absorption, *Res. Comm. Chem. Path. Pharmacol.*, 1979, **24**, 77.

129. Beckett, A.H., Important formulation factors influencing drug absorption in, *Drug Absorption*, Ed., Prescott, L.F. and Nimmo, W.S., MTP Press Ltd., Lancaster, 1979, 133.

130. Barr, W.H., Factors involved in the assessment of systemic or biologic availability of drug products, *Drug Inform Bull.*, 1969, **3**, 27.

131. Benet, L.Z., Biopharmaceutics as a basis for the design of drug products in, *Drug Design*, Vol. 4, Ed., Ariens, E.J., Academic Press, 1973.

132. Benet, L.Z., Input Factors as determinants of drug activitiy: Route, dose, dosage regimen and the drug delivery system in, *Principles and Techniques of Human Research and Therapeutics.*, Vol. 3, Ed., McMahan, F.G., Future Publishing Co., New York, 1974.

133. Ritschel, W.A., The scientific basis of bioavailability, *Labo-Pharma-Problems et Techniques*, 1978, **26**, 395.

134. Kawalek, J.C. and Andrews, A.W., The effects of solvents on drug metabolism *in vitro, Drug Metab. Dispos.*, 1980, **5**, 380.

135. Cambon, C., Fernandez. Y., Falzon, M. and Mitjavila, A.S., Variations of the digestive absorption kinetics of carbaryl with the nature of the vehicle, *Toxicology*, 1981, **22**, 45.

136. Bentley, E.W., Larthe, Y. and Taylor, A., The effect of particle size on the toxicity of a-napthyl thiourea (ANTO) to albino rats, *J. Hyg. Cambs.*, 1955, **53**, 328.

137. Fincher, J.H., Particle size of drugs and its relationship to absorption and activity, *J. Pharm. Sci.*, 1968, **57**, 1825.

138. Levy, G. and Juske, W.J., Effect of viscosity on drug absorption, *J. Pharm. Sci.*, 1965, **54**, 219.

139. Ritschel, W.A., Siegel, E.G. and Ring, D.E., Biopharmaceutical factors influencing LD_{50}: Pt. I Viscosity, *Arzneim - Forsch*, 1974, **24**, 907.

140. Shah, N.B. and Sheth, B.B., Effect of polymers on dissolution from drug suspensions, *J. Pharm. Sci.*, 1976, **65**, 1618.

141. Barzegar–Jalali, M. and Richards, J.H., The effect of various suspending agents on the bioavailabilies of aspirin and salicyclic acid in the rabbit, *Int. J. Pharmaceutics*, 1979, **3**, 133.

142. Barzegar–Jalali, M. and Richards, J.H., The effect of viscosity on the bio-

availability of nitrofurantoin from suspension dosage forms in the rats, *Int. J. Pharm. Tech. and Prod. Mfr.*, 1980, **1**, 22.

143. Eikholt, T.H. and White, W.F., The toxicity and absorption enhancing ability of surfactants, *Drug Stand.*, 1969, **28**, 154.

144. Scheuplein, R. and Ross, L., Effects of surfactants and solvents on the permeability of epidermis, *J. Soc. Cosmet. Chem.*, 1970, **21**, 858.

145. Creasy, N.H., Allenby, A.C. and Schock, C., Mechanism of action of accelerants, *Br. J. Derm.*, 1971, **85**, 368.

146. Spiegel, A.J. and Noteworthy, M.M., Use of non-aqueous solvents in parenteral solvents, *J. Pharm. Sci.*, 1963, **52**, 917.

147. Worthley, E.G. and Schott, C.D., Pharmacotoxic evaluation of nine vehicles administered intra-peritonealy to mice, *Lloydia*, 1966, **29**, 123.

148. Bartsch, W., Sponer, G., Dietman, K. and Fuchs, G., Acute toxicity of various solvents in the mouse and rat, *Arzneim – Forsch*, 1976, **26**, 158.

149. Drew, R. and Gram, T.E., Vehicle alteration of paraquat lethality in mice, *Tox. Appl. Pharmacol.*, 1975, **48**, 479.

150. Fletcher, J., Ethical considerations in biomedical research involving human beings, *Bull. Wld. Hlth. Org.*, 1977, **55** (Suppl. 2), 101.

151. Hayes, W.J., Jr., Ethical considerations involving studies of pesticides and other xenobiotics in man in, *Pesticides Chemistry: Human Welfare and the Environment*, Vol. 3, Eds., Miyamoto, J. and Kearney, P.C., Pergamon Press, 1983.

152. Brown, V.K., Avian toxicity tests with agricultural chemicals, in, *Proceedings of the European Society of Toxicology*, Karlova-Vary, Excerpta Medica International Congress Series No. 345, 1975, 125.

153. Stephenson, R.R., Aquatic toxicology of cypermethrin: I Acute toxicity to some freshwater fish and invertebrates in laboratory tests, *Aquatic Toxicology*, 1982, **2**, 175.

154. Brown, V.K., *Acute Toxicity in Theory and Practice*, John Wiley and Sons, 1980.

155. Brown, V.K., Acute toxicity testing in, *Animals and Alternatives in Toxicity Testing*, Eds., Ball, M., Riddell, R.J. and Worden, A.N., Academic Press, 1983.

156. Theil, H., *Principles of Econometrics*, John Wiley and Sons Inc., 1971.

157. Namba, T., Nolte, C.T., Jackrel, J. and Grob, D., Poisoning due to organophosphate insecticides: Acute and chronic manifestations, *Am. J. Med.*, 1971, **50**, 475.

158. Clark, G., Organophosphate insecticides and behaviour: A review, *Aerospace Med.*, 1971, **42**, 735.

159. Ludomirsky, A., Klein, H.O., Sarelli, P., Becker, B., Hoffman, S., Taitelman, U., Barzita, J., Lang, R., David, D., DiSegne, E. and Kaplinsky, E., Q-T prolongation and polymorphous ("Torsado de Pointes") ventricular arrhythmias associated with organophosphorus insecticide poisoning, *Am. J. Cardiol.*, 1982, **49**, 1654.

160. Fowler, J.S.L., Brown, J.S. and Bell, H.A., The rat toxicity screen, *Pharmac. Ther.*, 1979, **5**, 461.

161. Sperling, F. and McLaughlin, J.L., Biological parameters and the acute LD_{50} test, *J.A.O.A.C.*, 1976, **59**, 734.

162. Loomis, T.A., A review of the validity of presently accepted scientific standards in, *The Future of Animals, Cells, Models and Systems in Research, Development, Education and Testing* (Proceedings of a symposium), National Academy of Sciences – Washington DC, 1977.

163. Zbinden, G. and Flury-Roversi, M., Significance of the LD_{50} test for the toxicological evaluation of chemical substances, *Arch. Toxicol.*, 1981, **47**, 77.

164. Throdahl, M.C., The technical basis for decision making, *Chemistry and Industry*, 1 April 1978, 221.

165. Van Rossum, J.M., Van Lingen, G. and Burgers, J.P.T., Dose-dependent pharmacokinetics, *Pharmac. Ther.*, 1983, **21**, 77.

166. Molinengo, L., The curve doses vs. survival times in the evaluation of acute toxicity, *J. Pharm. Pharmacol.*, 1979, **31**, 343.

167. Puri, P.S. and Senturia, J., On a mathematical theory of quantal response assays in, *6th Berkeley Symposium on Mathematical Statistics and Probability*, Eds., Cann, Neyman and Scott, University of California Press, Berkeley and Los Angeles, 1972.

168. Waud, D.R., On biological assays involving quantal responses, *J. Pharmacol. exptl. Therap.*, 1972, **183**, 577.

169. Van Ryzin, J. and Rai, K., The use of quantal response data to make predictions in, *Developments in Toxicology and Environmental Science*, Vol. 6: The Scientific Basis of Toxicity Assessment, Ed., Witsch, H., Elsevier/North Holland Biomedical Press, 1980.

170. Hewlett, P.S. and Plackett, R.L., *The Interpretation of Quantal Responses in Biology*, Edward Arnold, 1979.

171. Hayes, W.J., Jr., The 90-dose LD_{50} and a chronicity factor as measures of toxicity, *Tox. Appl. Pharmacol.*, 1967, **11**, 327.

172. Trevan, J.W., The error of determination of toxicity, *Proc. Roy. Soc.*, 1927, **101** (Series B), 483.

173. Wright, S., A frequency curve adapted to variation in percentage occurrence, *J. Am. Stat. Assoc.*, 1926, **21**, 162.

174. Kuenen, D.J., Time–mortality curves and Abbott's correction in experiments with insecticides, *Acta Physiol. Pharmacol. Neerl.*, 1957, **6**, 179.

175. Zerva, G.N., Timoflievskaya, L.A., Stasenkova, K.P. and Bazarova, L.A., Utilization of time–effect curves in toxicological experiments, (in Russian), *Toxikol. Novykh. Promysch. Khim. Vesttchest.*, 1968, **10**, 5.

176. Jenkens, L.J., Jr., Jones, R.A. and Anderson, M.E., The use of mean survival time analysis in assessing toxic interactions, *Tox. Appl. Pharmacol.*, 1976, **37**, 129.

177. Brody, S., *Bioenergetics and Growth*, Hafner Publ. Co., New York, 1945.

178. Adolph, E.F., Quantitative relations in the physiological constitution of mammals, *Science*, 1949, **109**, 579.

179. Bailey, B.N., Observations on the validity of surface area evaluations of rats in the laboratory, *Texas Rpts. Biol. Med.*, 1962, **20**, 12.

180. Friis-Hansen, B., Body composition during growth, *Pediatrics*, 1971, **47**, 264.

181. Kleiber, M., Metabolic turnover rate: A physiological meaning of the metabolic rate per unit body weight, *J. Theor. Biol.*, 1975, **53**, 199.

182. Günther, B., *Fortschritte der Experimentellen und Theoretischen Biophysic*, Vol. 19: On Theories of Biological Similarity, Ed., Beier, W., Veb Georg Thieme, Leipzig, 1975.

183. Klippel, C.H., Surface area versus skin area, *New England J. Med.*, 1979, **301**, 730.

184. Economos, A.C., On structure and theories of basal metabolic rate, *J. Theor. Biol.*, 1979, **80**, 445.

185. Günther, B. and Morgado, E., Theory of biological similarity revisited, *J. Theor. Biol.*, 1982, **96**, 543.

186. Tanner, J.M., Fallacy of per-weight and per-surface area standards and their relation to spurious correlation, *J. Appl. Physiol.*, 1949, **2**, 1.

187. Weiss, M., Sziegozi, T.W. and Förster, W., Dependence of pharmacokinetic parameters on the body weight, *Int. J. Clin. Pharmacol.*, 1977 **15**, 572.

188. Pinkell, D., The use of body surface area as a criterion of drug dosage in cancer chemotherapy, *Cancer Res.*, 1958, **18**, 853.

189. Freireich, E.J., Gehan, E.A., Rall, D.P., Smidt, L.H. and Skipper, H.E., Quantitative comparison of toxicity of anti-cancer agents in mouse, rat, hamster, dog, monkey and man, *Cancer Chemother.*, 1966, **50**, 219.

190. Anderson, P.D. and Weber, L.J., Toxic response as a quantitative function of body size, *Tox. Appl. Pharmacol.*, 1975, **33**, 471.

191. Funaki, H., Drug toxicity (LD_{50}) and *dosis medicamentosa* for children in terms of body surface area and body weight, *J. Kyoto Pref. Univ. Med.*, 1974, **83**, 467.

192. Rall, D.P. and North, W.C., Toxicity of ANTU for the rat and its lack of dependence upon body weight, *Fed. Proc.*, 1952, **11**, 383.

193. Rall, D.P. and North, W.C., Consideration of dose–weight relationships, *Proc. Soc. exptl. Biol. Med.*, 1953, **83**, 825.

194. Angelakos, E.T., Lack of relationship between body weight and pharmacological effect exemplified by histamine toxicity in mice, *Proc. Soc. exptl. Biol. Med.*, 1960, **103**, 296.

195. Lamanna, C., The most poisonous poison, *Science*, 1959, **130**, 763.

196. Hanig, J.P. and Lamanna, C., Toxicity of botulinum toxin: A stoichometric model for the locus of its extraordinary potency and persistence at the neuromuscular junction, *J. Theor. Biol.*, 1979, **77**, 107.

197. Thonney, M.L., Touchberry, R.W., Goodrich, R.D. and Meiske, J.C., Re-evaluation of metabolic body weight, *J. Anim. Sci.*, 1974, **39**, 1002.

198. Bliss, C.I., The calculation of the dosage–mortality curve, *Ann. Appl. Biol.*, 1935, **22**, 134.

199. Litchfield, J.T., Jr., and Fertig, J.W., On a graphic solution of the dosage–effect curve, *Bull. John Hopkins Univ.*, 1941, **69**, 276.

200. Koch, A.L., The logarithm in biology: 1 Mechanisms generating the log-normal distribution exactly, *J. Theor. Biol.*, 1966, **12**, 296.

201. Koch, A.L., The logarithm in biology: 2 Distributions simulating the log-normal, *J. Theor. Biol.*, 1969, **23**, 251.

202. Gaddum, J.H., *Methods of Biological Assay Depending on a Quantal Response*, Med. Res. Cncl. Spec. Rpt. No. 183, 1933.

203. Finney, D.J., *Probit Analysis*, Cambridge University Press, Cambridge (3rd Edition), 1971.

204. Miller, L.C. and Tainter, M.L., Estimation of the LD_{50} and its error by means of logarithmic–probit graph paper, *Proc. Soc. exptl. Biol. Med.*, 1944, **57**, 261.

205. Litchfield, J.T., Jr., and Wilcoxon, F., A simplified method of evaluating dose–effects experiments, *J. Pharmacol. exptl. Therap.*, 1949, **96**, 99.

206. Fink, H. and Hund, G., Probitanalyse mittels programmgesteuerter rechenanlagen, *Arzneimittelforschung*, 1965, **15**, 624.

207. Rosiello, A.P., Essigmann, J.M. and Wogan, G.N., Rapid and accurate determination of the median lethal dose (LD_{50}) and its error with a small computer, *J. Toxicol. environ. Hlth.*, 1977, **3**, 797.

208. Thakur, A.K. and Fezio, W.L., A computer program for estimating LD_{50} and its confidence limits using modified Behrens-Reed-Muench cumulant method, *Drug Chem. Toxicol.*, 1981, **4**, 297.

209. Cook, D.A. and Bielkiequez, B., A computer-associated technique for analysis and comparison of dose-response curves, *J. Pharmacol. Methods*, 1983, **11**, 77.

210. Dunnett, C.W., Biostatistics in pharmacological testing in, *Selected Pharmacological Testing Methods*, Ed., Burger, A., Edward Arnold, 1968.

211. Cox, C.P., Statistical principles for the line of best fit, *Lab. Practice*, 1963, **12**, 733.

212. Gad, S.D. and Weil, C.S., Statistics for toxicologists in, *Principles and Methods of Toxicology*, Ed., A. Wallace Hayes, Raven Press, New York, 1982.

213. Weil, C.S., Statistics on safety factors and scientific judgement in the evaluation of safety for man, *Tox. Appl. Pharmacol.*, 1972a, **21**, 454.

214. Weil, C.S., Guidelines for experiments to predict the degree of safety of a material for man, *Tox. Appl. Pharmacol.*, 1972, **21**, 194.

215. Haley, T.J., Farmer, J.H., Dooley K.L., Harman, J.R. and Peoples, A., Determination of the LD_{01} and extrapolation of the LD_{001} for methyl-carbamate pesticides, *Europ. J. Toxicol.*, 1974, **7**, 152.

216. Haley, T.J., Harman, J.R., Dooley, K.L. and Uhler, R., Comparison of the LD_{01} of carbaryl and dichlorvos, *Fed. Proc.*, 1974, **33**, 230.

217. Haley, T.J., Farmer, J.H., Harman, J.R. and Dooley, K.L., Estimation of the LD_1 and extrapolation of the $LD_{0.1}$ for five organothiophosphate pesticides, *Europ. J. Toxicol.*, 1975, **8**, 229.

218. Haley, T.J., Farmer, J.H., Harman, J.R. and Dooley, K.L. Estimation of the $LD_{0.1}$ for five organophosphate pesticides, *Arch. Toxicol.*, 1975, **34**, 104.

219. Brown, V.K.H., Ferrigan, L.W. and Stevenson, D.E., The acute toxicity and skin irritant properties of tropilidene (cyclohepta-1,3,5-triene), *Ann. Occup. Hyg.*, 1967, **10**, 123.

220. Karber, G., Beitrog zue kollectiven behandlung pharmakologische Reihen-versuche, *Arch. exptl. Path. Pharmakol.*, 1931, **162**, 480.

221. Chanter, D.O. and Heywood, R., The LD_{50} test; Some consideration of precision, *Tox. Letters.*, 1982, **10**, 303.

222. Bross, I., Estimates of the LD_{50}: A critique, *Biometrics*, 1950, **6**, 413.

223. Armitage, P. and Allen, I., Methods of estimating the LD_{50} in quantal response data, *J. Hyg.*, 1950, **48**, 298.

224. Livshits, P.Z., On the estimation of the median lethal dose (in Russian), *Farmakol. Tokikol.*, 1966, **29**, 113.

225. Knudsen, L.F. and Curtis, J.M., The use of angular transformation in biological assays, *J. Am. Statist. Assoc.*, 1947, **42**, 282.

226. Berkson, J., Application of the logistic function to bio-assay, *J. Am. Statist. Assoc.*, 1944, **39**, 357.

227. Rybach, E.I., Lisunkin, Y.I. and Kalinin, O.M., The determination of the 50% and other doses by a method of statistical approximation (in Russian), *Farmakol. Toxicol.*, 1966, **29**, 368.

228. Thompson, W.R. and Weil, C.S., On the construction of tables of moving-average interpolation, *Biometrics*, 1952, **8**, 51.

229. Weil, C.S., Tables for convenient calculation of median-effective dose (LD_{50} or ED_{50}) and instructions in their use, *Biometrics*, 1952, **8**, 249.

230. Weil, C.S., Economical LD_{50} and slope determinations, *Drug Chem. Toxicol.*, 1983, **6**, 595.

231. Aitchison, J. and Silvey, S.D., The generalization of probit analysis to the case of multiple responses, *Biometrika*, 1951, **44**, 131.

232. Ashford, J.R., An approach to the analysis of data for semi-quantal responses in biological assay, *Biometrics*, 1959, **15**, 573.

233. Gurland, J., Lee, I. and Dahm, P.A., Polychotomous quantal response in biological assay, *Biometrics.*, 1960, **16**, 382.

234. Gardock, J.F., Yelnosky, J., Kuchn, W.F. and Gunster, J.C., A study of the interaction of nalorphine with fentamyl and Innovar, *Tox. Appl. Pharmacol.*, 1964, **6**, 593.

235. Gardock, J.F., Schuler, M.E. and Goldstein, L., Reconsideration of the central nervous system pharmacology of amphetamine: I Toxicty in grouped and isolated mice, *Tox. Appl. Pharmacol.*, 1966, **8**, 550.

236. George, D.J. and Wolf, H.H., Dose–lethality curves for d-amphetamine in isolated and aggregated mice, *Life Sciences*, 1966, **5**, 1583.

237. Zavon, M.R., Interactions, *Bio Science*, 1969, **19**, 892.
238. Stockley, I., *Drug Interactions*, The Pharmaceutical Press, London, 1977.
239. Schaefer, H., Zesch, A. and Stüttgen, G., *Skin Permeability*, Springer-Verlag, 1982.
240. Welling, P.G., Influence of food and diet in gastro-intestinal drug absorption: A review, *J. Pharmacokinetic. Biopharm.*, 1979, **5**, 291.
241. Ferguson, H.C., Dilution of dose and acute oral toxicity, *Tox. Appl. Pharmacol.*, 1962, **4**, 759.
242. Borowitzy, J.L., Moore, P.F., Yim, K.W. and Mija, T.S., Mechanism of enhanced drug effects produced by dilution of the oral dose, *Tox. Appl. Pharmacol.*, 1971, **19**, 164.
243. Munro, J.B., Ostler, D.C., Machin, A.F. and Quick, M.P., Suspected poisoning by pentachlorophenol in sawdust, *Vet. Rec.*, 1977, **101**, 525.
244. Taylor, D., Dieldrin-poison threat that won't go away, *British Farm and Stockbreeder*, 19 August 1978, 22.
245. Dubois, K.P., Potentiation of the toxicity of insecticidal organic phosphates. *Arch. industr. Hlth.*, 1958, **18**, 488.
246. Murphy, S.D., Toxic interactions with dermal exposure to organophosphate insecticides in, *Mechanisms of Toxicity and Hazard Evaluation*, Ed., Holmstedt, B., Lauwerys, R., Mercier, M. and Roberfroid, M., Elsevier/North Holland Biomedical Press, Amsterdam, 1980.
247. Murphy, S.D., Assessment of the potential for toxic interactions among environmental pollutants in, *The Principles and Methods in Modern Toxicology*, Eds., Galli, C.L., Murphy, S.D. and Paoletti, R., Elsevier/North Holland Biomedical Press, Oxford, 1980.
248. Rosenberg, P. and Coon, J.M., Increase of hexabarbital sleeping time by certain anticholinesterases, *Proc. Soc. exptl. Biol. Med.*, 1958, **98**, 650.
249. Murphy, S.D., Mechanism of pesticide interactions in vertebrates, *Residue Revs.*, 1969, **25**, 201.
250. Stevens, J.T., Stitzer, R.E. and McPhillips, J.J., Effects of anticholinesterase insecticides on hepatic microsomal metabolism, *J. Pharmacol. exptl. Therap.*, 1972, **181**, 576.
251. Cohen, S.D., Mechanisms of toxicological interactions involving organophosphate insecticides, *Fund. Appl. Toxicol.*, 1984, **4**, 315.
252. Robinson, F.R., Harper, D.T., Jr., and Kaplam, H.P., Comparison of strains of rats exposed to oxygen and various pressures, *Lab. Anim. Care.*, 1967, **17**, 433.
253. Loewe, S., Coalitive actions of combined drugs, *J. Pharmacol. exptl. Ther.*, 1938, **63**, 24.
254. Loewe, S., Randbemerkungen zur quantitativen pharmakologie der kombinationen, *Arzneim – Forsch*, 1959, **9**, 449.
255. Ellin, R.J. and Wills, J.H., Oximes antagonistic to inhibitors of cholinesterase Pt 1, *J. Pharm. Sci.*, 1964a, **53**, 995.
256. Ellin, R.J. and Wills, J.H., Oximes antagonistic to inhibitors of cholinesterase Pt 2, *J. Pharm. Sci.*, 1964b, **53**, 4432.
257. Plackett, R.L., Theoretical aspect of the action of mixtures, *Chemistry and Industry*, 1 August 1981, 528.
258. Plackett, R.L. and Hewlett, P.S., Statistical aspects of the independent joint action of poisons, particularly insecticides, *Ann. Appl. Biol.*, 1948, **35**, 347.
259. Plackett, R.L. and Hewlett, P.S., Quantal responses to mixtures of poisons, *J. Roy. Statist. Soc.*, 1952, **14**, (Series B), 141.
260. Landahl, H.D., Theoretical considerations on potentiation in drug interaction, *Bull. Math. Biophys.*, 1958, **20**, 1–23.

261. Ashford, J.R., Quantal responses to mixtures of poisons under conditions of simple similar action – the analysis of uncontrolled data, *Biometrika*, 1958, **45**, 74.

262. Ashford, J.R., Biological and mathematical models, *Chemistry and Industry*, 1 August 1981, 521.

263. Ashford, J.R., General models for the joint action of mixtures, *Biometrics*, 1981b, **37**, 457.

264. Ashford, J.R. and Cobby, J.M., A system of models for the action of drugs applied singly or jointly to biological organisms, *Biometrics*, 1974, **30**, 11.

265. Ashford, J.R. and Smith, C.S., A general system of models for the action of mixtures of drugs in biological assay, *Biometrika*, 1964, **51**, 413.

266. Ashford, J.R. and Smith, C.S., An alternative system for the classification of mathematical models for quantal responses to mixtures of drugs in biological assay, *Biometrics*, 1965, **21**, 181.

267. Kagan, Y.S., Vojtento, Q.A., Svetlij, S.S. and Zlatjen, Z., A method for the quantitative evaluation of combined and complex pesticide effects on organisms in, *Pesticides – Environmental Quality and Safety* Supply. Vol. III, Ed., Coulston, F., Thieme, Stuttgart, 1975.

268. Schaeffer, D.J., Glave, W.R. and Janardan, K.G., Multivariate statistical methods in toxicology: III Specifying joint toxic interaction using multiple regression analysis, *J. Tox. Environ. Hlth.*, 1982, **9**, 705.

269. Sheldon, D.W. and Weber, L.J., Quantification of the joint effects of mixtures of hepatotoxic agents: Evaluation of a theoretical model in mice, *Environ. Res.*, 1981, **26**, 33.

270. Ball, W.S., The toxicological basis of threshold limit values: 4 Theoretical approach to prediction of toxicity of mixtures, Am. Industr. Hyg. Assoc. J., 1959, **20**, 257.

271. Rothman, K.J., Synergy and antagonism in cause–effect relationship, *Am. J. Epidemiol.*, 1974, **99**, 385.

272. Alabaster, J.S., Joint action of mixtures of toxicants on aquatic organisms, *Chemistry and Industry*, 1 August 1981, 529.

273. Könemann, H., Fish toxicity tests with mixtures of more than two chemicals: A proposal for a quantitative approach and experimental results, *Toxicology*, 1981, **19**, 229.

274. Ariens, E.J., van Rossum, J.M. and Simonis, A.M., Affinity, intrinsic activity and drug interaction, *Pharmacol. Revs.*, 1957, **9**, 218.

275. Schand, D.G., Mitchell, J.R. and Oates, J.A., Pharmacokinetic drug interactions in, *Handbuch der experimentellen Pharmakologie (Concepts in Biochemical Pharmacology)* Pt. 3, Eds., Gillette, J.R. and Mitchell, J.R., Springer-Verlag, 1975.

276. Gillette, J.R. and Mitchell, J.R., Drug actions and interactions; Theoretical considerations in, *Handbuch der experimentellen Pharmakologie (Concepts in Biochemical Pharmacology)* Pt 3, Eds., Gillette, J.R. and Mitchell, J.R., Springer-Verlag, 1975.

277. Ioannides, C., Drug interactions in, *Clinical Implications of Drug Use*, Vol. II, Ed., Basu, T.K., CRC Press Inc. Boca Raton, 1980.

278. Marchant, B., Pharmacokinetic drug interactions of non-steroidal anti-inflammatory agents, *Chemistry and Industry*, 1 August 1981, 534.

279. Stahl, P.H., The problems of drug interactions with excipients in, *Towards Better Safety of Drugs and Pharmaceutical Products*, Ed., Breimer, D.D., Elesvier/North Holland Biomedical Press, 1980.

280. Griffin, J.P., Drug interactions occurring during absorption from the gastro-intestinal tract, *Pharmac. Ther.*, 1981, **15**, 79.

281. Anon, Adverse interactions of drugs, *The Medical Letter on Drugs and Therapeutics.*, 1981, **23**, 17.

282. Sumerford, W.T., Review of synergism among halogen containing insecticides and halogen containing synergists, *J. Agr. Fd. Chem.*, 1954, **2**, 310.

283. Keplinger, M.L. and Deichmann, W.B., Acute toxicity of combinations of pesticides, *Tox. Appl. Pharmacol.*, 1967, **10**, 586.

284. Wysocka-Paruszewska, B., Osicka, A., Brzezinski, J. and Gradowska, I. An evaluation of the toxicity of thiuram in combination with other pesticides, *Arch. Toxicol.* (Suppl. 4), 1980, 449.

285. Clausing, P. and Bieleke, R., Aspects of methodology employed in the investigation of combined chemical effects on acute oral toxicity, *Arch. Toxicol.* (Suppl. 4), 1980, 394.

286. De Jongh, S.E., Isoboles in, *Quantitative Methods in Pharmacology*, Ed., de Jongh, H., North Holland Publishing Co., Amsterdam, 1961.

287. Loewe, S., The problem of synergism and antagonism of combined drugs, *Arzneim. – Forsch.*, 1953, **3**, 285.

288. Loewe, S., Antagomisms and antagonists, *Pharmacol. Revs.*, 1957, **9**, 237.

289. Smyth, H.F., Jr., Weil, C.S., West, J.S. and Carpenter, C.P., An explanation of joint toxic action: Twenty-seven industrial chemicals intubated in rats in all possible pairs, *Tox. Appl. Pharmacol.*, 1969, **14**, 340.

290. Dayan, A.D., Uses and limitations of primates in the evaluation of drug efficacy and safety, *J. Roy. Soc. Med.*, 1978, **71**, 691.

291. Dayan, A.D., The relative worth of animal testing in, *Risk–Benefit Analysis in Drug Research*, Ed., Cavalla, J.F., MTP Press Ltd., 1981, Lancaster.

292. Dedrick, R.L., Animal scale-up, *J. Pharmacokin. Biopharm.*, 1973, **1**, 435.

293. Dedrick, R.L. and Bischoff, K.B., Species similarities in pharmacokinetics, *Fed. Proc.*, 1980, **39**, 54.

294. Ryder, R.D., *Victims of science – the use of animals in research*, David-Poynter, London, 1975.

295. Bankowski, Z. and Gutteridge, F., Medical ethics and human research, *World Health*, 1982, (issue for November 1982), 10–13.

296. Smith, C.C., Value of non-human primates in predicting disposition of drugs in man. *Ann. N.Y. Acad. Sci.*, 1969, **162**, 604.

297. Reynolds, H.H., Non-human primates in the study of toxicological effects on the central nervous system: A Review, *Ann. N.Y. Acad. Sci.*, 1969, **162**, 617.

298. Coulston, F. and Serrone, D.M., The comparative approach to the role of non-human primates in evaluation of drug toxicity in man: A Review, *Ann. N.Y. Acad. Sci.*, 1969, **162**, 681.

299. Hawkins, D.R., The use of non-human primates in models for the metabolism of pesticides and xenobiotics in man in, *Pesticide Chemistry: Human Welfare and the Environment*, Vol. 3, Eds., Miyamoto, J. and Kearney, P.C., Pergamon Press, 1983.

300. Litchfield, J.T., Jr. Symposium on clinical drug evaluation and human pharmacology: VXI evaluation of the safety of new drugs by means of tests in animals, *Clin. Pharmacol. Therap.*, 1962, **3**, 665.

301. Van Noordwijk, J., Communication between the experimental animal and the pharmacologist, *Statist. Neerl.*, 1964, **18**, 403.

302. Perlman, P.L., Transfer of animal pharmacology and toxicology data to man, *Drug. Info. Bull.*, 1970, **4**, 7.

303. Baker, S.B. de C. and Davey, D.G., The predictive value for man of toxicological tests of drugs in laboratory animals, *Br. Med. Bull.*, 1970, **26**, 208.

304. Krasovskij, G.N. and Sobinyakova, O.R., Comparative sensitivity of man and animals to the action of various substances according to indices of acute toxicity. (in Russian), *Gig. Sanit.*, 1970, **35**, 29.

305. Smith, C.G., Poutsiaka, J.W. and Schreiber, E.C., Problems in 1973, predicting drug effects across species lines, *J. Int. Med. Res.*, 1973, **1**, 489.

306. Gillette, J.R., Application of pharmacokinetic principles in the extrapolation of animal data to humans, *Clin. Tox.*, 1976, **9**, 709.

307. Krasovskij, G.N., Extrapolation of experimental data from animals to man, *Environ. Hlth. Perspect.*, 1976, **13**, 51.

308. Coid, C.R., Tests in laboratory animals – are they valid for man? *J. Roy. Soc. Med.*, 1978, **71**, 675.

309. Kenaga, E.E., Test organisms and methods useful for early assessment of acute toxicity of chemicals, *Environ. Sci. Technol.*, 1978, **12**, 1322.

310. Reichsman, F.P. and Calabrese, E.J., Animals extrapolations in environmental health: its theoretical basis and practical applications, *Revs. Environ. Hlth.*, 1978, **3**, 60.

311. Mondino, A., The choice of animal species in experimental toxicology in, *The Principles and Methods in Modern Toxicology*, Eds., Galli, C.L., Murphy, S.D. and Paoletti, R., Elsevier/North Holland Biomedical press, 1980.

312. Oser, B.L., The rat as a model for human toxicology evaluation, *J. Tox. Environ. Hlth.*, 1981, **8**, 521.

313. Doull, J., Assessing pesticide toxicity in man and correlations with laboratory animal studies in, *Pesticide Chemistry: Human Welfare and the Environment*, Vol. 3, Eds., Miyamato, J. and Kearney, P.C., Pergamon Press, 1983.

314. Calabrese, E.J., *Principles of animal extrapolation*, John Wiley and Sons, 1983.

315. Borison, H.L. and Wang, S.C., Physiology and pharmacology of vomitting, *Pharmacol. Revs.*, 1953, **5**, 193.

316. Hutson, D.G. and Hathway, D.E., Toxic effects of chlorfenvinphos in dogs and rats, *Biochem. Pharmacol.*, 1967, **16**, 949.

317. Schantz, E.J. and Scott, A.B., Use of crystalline-type A botulinum toxin in medical research in *Biomedical Aspects of Botulism*, Ed., Lewis, G.E., Jr., Academic Press, 1981, 143.

318. Cunha, T.J., *Swine feeding and nutrition*, Academic Press, 1977.

319. Wiberg, G.S., Colderwell, B.B. and Trenholm, H.L., The development of a systematic method for toxicological research using an integrated multidisciplinary approach. *Clin. Toxicol.*, 1971, **4**, 79.

320. Kulkarni, A.P. and Hodgson, E., Comparative toxicology in, *Introduction to Biochemical Toxicology*, Eds., Hodgson, E. and Guthrie, F.E., Blackwell Scientific Publications, 1980.

321. Koppanyi, T. and Avery, M.A., Species differences and the clinical trial of a new drug: A Review, *Clin. Pharmacol. Ther.*, 1966, **7**, 250.

322. Maibach, H.I., Feldmann, R.J., Milby, T.H. and Serat, W.F., Regional variation in percutaneous penetration in man, *Arch. Environ. Hlth.*, 1971 **23**, 208.

323. Wester, R.C. and Noonan, P.K., Relevance of animal models for percutaneous absorption, *Int. J. Pharmaceut.*, 1980, **7**, 99.

324. Sanockij, I.V., Methods for determining toxicity and hazards of chemicals quoted in, *Principles and Methods for Evaluating the Toxicity of Chemicals Part 1 (Environmental Health Criteria 6)*, World Health Organisation – Geneva, 1978.

325. Brown, R.A., Jr., and Schanker, L.S., Species comparison of aerosolized drug absorption from the lung, *The Toxicologist*, 1982, **2**, 224.

326. Etkin, N.L., Mahoney, J.R., Forsthoefel, M.W., Eckman, J.R., McSwigan, J.D., Gillum, R.F. and Eaton, J.W., Racial differences in hypertension-associated red cell sodium permeability, *Nature*, 1982, **297**, 588.

327. Kalow, W., *Pharmacogenetics – Heredity and the Response to Drugs*, W.B. Saunders Co., Philadelphia and London, 1962.

328. Kalow, W., Dose–response relationship and genetic variation, *Ann. N.Y. Acad. Sci.*, 1965, **123**, 212.

329. Brown, A.M., Pharmacogenetics of the mouse, *Lab. Anim. Care*, 1965, **15**, 111.

330. Guthrie, F.E., Monroe, R.J. and Abernathy, C.O., Response of the laboratory mouse to selection for resistance to insecticides, *Tox. Appl. Pharmacol.*, 1971, **18**, 92.

331. Webb, R.E., Hartgrove, R.W., Randolph, W.C., Petrella, V.J. and Horsfall, F., Jr., Toxicity studies in endrin-susceptible and resistant strains of pine mice, *Tox. Appl. Pharmacol.*, 1973, **25**, 42.

332. Hill, R.N., Clemens, T.L., Liv, D.K. to Vesell, E.S., Genetic control of chloroform toxicity in mice, *Science*, 1975, **190**, 159.

333. Lang, C.M. and Vesell, E.S., Environmental and genetic factors affecting laboratory animals: Impact on biomedical research, *Fed. Proc.*, 1976, **35**, 1123.

334. Hilado, C.J. and Furst, A., Reproducibility of toxicity test data as a function of mouse strain, animal lot and operator, *J. Combust. Toxicol.*, 1978, **5**, 75.

335. Haley, T.J., Dooley, K.L. and Harmon, J.R., Acute oral toxicity of *N*-2-fluorenylacetamide (2-FAA) in several strains of mice, *Proc. Soc. exptl. Biol. Med.*, 1973, **143**, 1117.

336. Miura, K., Ino, T. and Izuka, S., Comparison of the susceptibilities to the acute toxicity of BHC in strains of experimental mice (in Japanese), *Jikken Dobutsu*, 1974, **2**, 198.

337. Chapman, D.E. and Schiller, C.M., Comparative toxicity of 2,3,7,8-tetrachloro-dibenzo-*p*-dioxin (TCDD), *The Toxicologist*, 1984, **4**, 187.

338. Rack, G.J., Biological variability: Precision in bio-medical research in *The Future of Animals, Cells, Models and Systems in Research, Development, Education and Testing*, National Academy of Sciences – Washington DC, 1977.

339. Rowland, M., Intra-individual variability in pharmacokinetics, in *Towards Better Safety of Drugs and Pharmaceutical Products*, Ed., Breimer, D.D., Elsevier/North Holland Biomedical Press, 1980.

340. Brown, V.K.H., Acute toxicity testing: A critique in *Testing for Toxicity*, Ed., Gorrod, J.W., Taylor and Francis, London, 1981.

341. Basu, T.K., Pharmacological response as a function of age in, *Clinical Implications of Drug Use*, Vol. II, Ed., Basu, T.K., CRC Press Inc., Boca Raton, 1980.

342. Mann, D.E., Jr., Biological ageing and its modification of drug activity, *J. Pharm. Sci.*, 1965, **54**, 499.

343. Stave, V., Age-dependent changes of metabolism: I Studies of enzyme patterns of rabbit organs, *Biol. Neonat*, 1964, **6**, 128.

344. Hommes, F.A. and Wilmink, C.W., Development changes of glycolytic enzymes in rat brain, liver and skeletal muscle, *Biol. Neonat*, 1968, **12**, 181.

345. Spencer, R.P., Variation of intestinal activity with age: A review, *Yale J. Biol. Med.*, 1964, **37**, 105.

346. Khera, K.S. and Clegg, D.J., Perinatal toxicity of pesticides, *J. Canad. Med. Assoc.*, 1969, **100**, 167.

347. Maxwell, G.M., *Principles of Paediatric Pharmacology*, Croom Helm, 1984.

348. Valdes-Dapena, M.A. and Arey, J.B., Boric acid poisoning: Three fatal cases with pancreatic inclusions and a review of the literature, *J. Paediatrics*, 1962, **61**, 531.

349. Wong, L.C., Heimbach, M.D., Truscott, D.R. and Duncan, B.D., Boric acid poisoning: Report of 11 cases, *Canad. Med. Assoc. J.*, 1964, **90**, 1018.

350. Curley, A., Hawk, R.E., Kimbrough, R.D., Nathenson, G. and Finberg, L.,

Dermal absorption of hexachlorophane in infants, *The Lancet*, i., 1971, 296.

351. Lockhart, J.D., How toxic is hexachlorophane? *Pediatrics*, 1972, **50**, 29.

352. Nyhan, W.L., Toxicity of drugs in the neonatal period, J. Pediat., 1961, **59**, 1.

353. Yearly, R.A., Benish, R.A. and Finkelstein, M., Acute toxicity of drugs in newborn animals, *J. Pediat.*, 1966, **69**, 663.

354. Jusko, W.J., Pharmacokinetic principles in pediatric pharmacology, *Ped. Clin. North America*, 1972, **19**, 81.

355. Hilligoss, D.M., Neonatal pharmacokinetics in, *Applied Pharmacokinetics*, Eds., Evans, W.E., Schentag, J.J. and Jusoko, W.J., Applied Therapeutics Inc., San Francisco, 1980.

356. Goldenthal, E.I., A compilation of LD_{50} values in newborn and adult animals, *Tox. Appl. Pharmacol.*, 1971, **18**, 185.

357. Lu, F.C., Jessup, D.C. and Lavallee, A., Toxicity of pesticides in young versus adult rats, *Fd. Cosmet. Toxicol.*, 1965, **3**, 591.

358. Harbison, R.D., Comparative toxicity of some selected pesticides in neonatal and adult rats, *Tox. Appl. Pharmacol.*, 1974, **32**, 443.

359. Harbison, R.D. and Koshakij, R.P., Studies on the mechanism of increased susceptibility of the newborn to parathion toxicity, *Fed. Proc.*, 1975, **34**, 245.

360. Benke, G.M. and Murphy, S.D., The influence of age in the toxicity and metabolism of methylparathion and parathion in mice and female rats, *Tox. Appl. Pharmacol.*, 1975, **31**, 254.

361. Kupferberg, H.J. and Way, E.L., Pharmacologic basis for the increased sensitivity of the newborn rat to morphine, *J. Pharmacol. exptl. Ther.*, 1963, **141**, 105.

362. Brus, R. and Herman, Z.S., Acute toxicities of adrenalin, noradrenalin and actylcholine in adult and neonatal mice, *Dissert. Pharm. Pharmacol.*, 1971, **23**, 435.

363. Greengard, J., Iron poisoning in children, *Clin. Toxicol.*, 1975, **8**, 575.

364. Gädeke, R., Ein medizingeschichteiches panorama der Akuten Eisenvergiftung, *Klin. Pädiat.*, 1979, **191**, 442.

365. James, T.C. and Kanungo, M.S., Alternatives in atropine sites of the brain of rats as a function of age, *Biochem. Biophys. Res. Comms.*, 1976, **72**, 170.

366. Kato, R. and Takanaka, A., Metabolism of drugs in old rats: II Metabolism *in vivo* and effect of drugs in old rats, *Jap. J. Pharmac.*, 1968, **18**, 399.

367. Lasagna, L., Drug effects as modified by ageing, *J. Chronic. Dis.*, 1956, **3**, 567.

368. Bender, A.D., A pharmacodynamic basis for changes in drug activity associated with ageing in the adult, *Exp. Geriat.*, 1965, **1**, 237.

369. Bender, A.D., Pharmacologic aspects of ageing: A survey of the effect of increasing age on drug activity in adults, *J. Amer. Geriat. Soc.*, 1964, **12**, 114.

370. Salmon, T.P. and Marsh, R.E., Age as a factor in rodent susceptibility to rodenticides – A review in, *Vertebrate Pest Control and Management Materials* (ASTM STP 680), Ed., Beck, J.R., American Society for Testing and Materials, Philadelphia, 1979, 84.

371. Rath, S. and Misra, B.N., Relative toxicity of dichlorvos (DDVP) to *Tilapia mossambica*, (Peters) of 3 different age groups, *Exp. Geriat.*, 1979, **14**, 307.

372. Hudson, R.G., Tucker, R.K. and Haegele, M.A., Effect of age on sensitivity: Acute oral toxicity of 14 pesticides to mallard duck of several ages, *Tox. Appl. Pharmacol.*, 1972, **22**, 556.

373. Noordhoek, J. and Rümke, C.L., Sex differences in the rate of drug metabolism in mice, *Arch. Int. Pharmacodyn.*, 1969, **182**, 401.

374. Rowe, F.P. and Redfern, R., The effect of sex and age on the response to warfarin in a non-inbred strain of mice, *J. Hyg. Camb.*, 1967, **65**, 55.

375. Gaines, T.B., Acute toxicity of pesticides, *Tox. Appl. Pharmacol.*, 1969, **14**, 515.

376. Steen, J.A., Hanneman, G.D., Nelson, P.L. and Folk, E.D., Acute toxicity of mevinphos to gerbils, *Tox. Appl. Pharmacol.*, 1976, **35**, 195.

377. Schenkman, J.B., Frey, I., Remmer, H. and Estabrook, R.W., Sex differences in drug metabolism by rat liver microsomes, *Mol. Pharmacol.*, 1967, **3**, 5.

378. Kato, R., Sex-related différences in drug metabolism, *Drug Metab. Revs.*, 1974, **3**, 1.

379. Baty, J.D., Species, strains and sex differences in metabolism in, *Foreign Compound Metabolism in Mammals*, Ed., Hathway, D.E., The Chemical Society, London, 1979.

380. Kato, R., Takanaka, A. and Takayanagi, M., Studies on mechanism of sex differences in drug-oxidising activity of liver microsomes, *Jap. J. Pharmac.*, 1968, **18**, 482.

381. Gregory, M., Monro, A., Quinton, M. and Woolhouse, N., The acute toxicity of oxamniquine in rats; sex-dependent hepatotoxicity, *Arch. Toxicol.*, 1983, **54**, 247.

382. Toothaker, R.D. and Welling, P.G., The effect of food on drug bioavailability, *Ann. Rev. Pharmacol. Toxicol.*, 1980, **20**, 173.

383. Komuro, T., Kitazawa, S. and Sezaki, H., Fasting and the volume of drug distribution in the rat, *Chem. Pharm. Bull.*, 1975, **23**, 909.

384. Kitazawa, S. and Komuro, T., Effect of fasting on body fluids and intestinal drug absorption in rats, *Chem. Pharm. Bull.*, 1977, **25** 327.

385. Kast, A. and Nishikawa, J., The effect of fasting on acute toxicity of drugs in rats and mice, *Lab Anim.*, 1981, **15**, 359.

386. Achord, J.L., Acute effects of fasting on gastro-intestinal structure and function, *Med. Times*, 1967, **95**, 441.

387. Freedland, R.A., Effect of progressive starvation on rat liver enzymes activities, *J. Nutr.*, 1967, **91**, 489.

388. Birt, D.F. and Schuldt, G.H., Dietary amino-acids and hepatic microsomal drug metabolism in Syrian hamsters, *Drug–Nutrient Interaction*, 1982, **1**, 177.

389. Campbell, T.C., Modern concepts in nutritional status and foreign compound toxicity in, *Advances in Modern Toxicology*, Vol. 1, Pt. 1 (New Concepts in Safety Evaluation), Eds., Mehlman, M.A., Shapiro, R.E. and Blumenthal. H., Hemisphere Publishing Corpn., Washington and London, 1976.

390. Basu, T.K., Nutritional status and drug therapy in, *Clinical Implications of Drug Use.*, Vol. II, Ed., Basu, T.K., CRC Press Inc., Baca Raton., 1980.

391. Kaloyanova, F. and Tasheva, M., Effect of protein malnutrition on the toxicity of pesticides in, *Pesticide Chemistry: Human Welfare and the Environment*, Vol. 3, Eds., Miyamoto, J. and Kearney, P.C., Pergamon Press, 1983.

392. Charbonneau, G.M. and Munro, E.C., Dietary factors affecting pesticide toxicity in *Pesticide Chemistry: Human Welfare and the Environment*, Vol. 3, Eds., Miyamoto, J. and Kearney, P.C., Pergamon Press, 1983.

393. Boyd, E.M., *Predictive Toxicometrics.*, Scientechnica Publishers Ltd., Bristol, 1972.

394. Halberg, F., Chronobiology, *Ann. Rev. Physiol.*, 1969, **31**, 675.

395. Bünning, E., *The Physiological Clock: Circadian Rhythms and Biological Chronometry.*, The English Universities Press Ltd., London, (3rd Edition), 1973.

396. Scheving, L.E. and Pavey, J.E., Chronobiology – its implications for clinical medicine in, *Annual Reports in Medicinal Chemistry*. Vol. II, Editor-in-Chief: Clark, F.H., Academic Press, 1976.

397. Stupfel, M., Biorhythms in toxicology and pharmacology: I Generalities, ultradian and circadian biorhythms, *Biomedicine*, 1975, **22**, 18.
398. Martinez-O'Ferrall, J.A., Circadian rhythms, *J. Occup. Med.*, 1968, **10**, 205.
399. Davis, W.M. and Webb, O.L., A circadian rhythm of chemo-convulsive response thresholds in mice, *Med. exp.*, 1963, **9**, 263.
400. Carlsson, A. and Serin, F., Time of day as a factor influencing the toxicity of nikethamide, *Acta Pharmacol.*, 1950, **6**, 181.
401. Carlsson, A. and Serin, F., The toxicity of nikethamide at different times of the day, *Acta Pharmacol.*, 1950, **6**, 187.
402. Luthra, R., Kyle, G. and Bruckner, J.V., The effect of time of dosing on chemical toxicity, *The Toxicologist*, 1982, **2**, 177.
403. Radzialowski, F.M. and Bousquet, W.F., Circadian rhythm in hepatic drug metabolizing activity in the rat, *Life Sciences*, 1967, **6**, 2545.
404. Radzialowski, F.M. and Bousquet, W.F., Daily rhythmic variation in hepatic drug metabolism in the rat and mouse, *J. Pharmacol. exp. Ther.*, 1968, **163**, 229.
405. Jori, A.F., Disalle, E. and Santini, V., Daily rhythmic variations and liver drug metabolism in rats, *Biochem. Pharmacol.*, 1971, **20**, 2965.
406. Lake, B.G., Tredger, J.M., Burke, M.D., Chakraborty, J. and Bridges, J.W., The circadian variation of hepatic microsomal drug and steroid metabolism in the golden hamster, *Chem. Biol. Interact.*, 1976, **12**, 81.
407. Tredger, J.M. and Chharbra, R.S., Circadian variations in microsomal drug metabolizing enzyme activities in rat and rabbit tissues, *Xenobiotic*, 1977, **7**, 481.
408. Schnell, R.C., Bozigian, H.P., Davies, M.H., Merrick, B.A. and Johnson, K.C., Circadian rhythm in aceaminophen toxicity: role of non-protein sulphydryls, *Tox. Appl. Pharmacol.*, 1983, **71**, 353.
409. Birt, D.F. and Schuldt, G.H., Dietary amino acids and hepatic microsomal drug metabolism in Syrian hamsters, *Drug–Nutrient Interactions.*, 1982, **1**, 177.
410. Birt, D.F. and Hines, L.A., Modification of circadian rhythms of drug metabolism in the Syrian hamster, *Drug–Nutrient Interactions*, 1982, **1**, 143.
411. Reinberg, A. and Halbert, F., Circadian chronopharmacology, *Ann. Rev. Pharmacol.*, 1971, **11**, 455.
412. Sturtevant, F.M., Sturtevant, R.P., Scheving, L.E. and Pavly, J.E., Chronopharmacokinetics of ethanol, *N.S. Arch. Pharmacol.*, 1976, **293**, 203.
413. Elsmore, T.F., Circadian susceptibility to soman poisoning, *Fund. Appl. Toxicol.*, 1981, **1**, 238.
414. Wolfe, G.W. and Schnell, R.C., Influence of hormonal factors on daily variations in hepatic drug metabolism in male rats, *J. Interdiscip. Cycle Res.*, 1979, **10**, 173.
415. Kato, R., Onoda, K-I and Takanaka, A., Species differences in the effect of morphine administration or adrenalectomy on the substrate interactions with cytochrome P-450 and drug oxidations by liver microsomes, *Biochem. Pharmacol.*, 1971, **20**, 1093.
416. Bousquet, W.F., Rupe, B.D. and Miya, T.S., Endocrine modification of drug responses, in the rat, *J. Pharm. exptl. Ther.*, 1965, **147**, 376.
417. Civen, M. and Brown, C.B., The effect of organophosphate insecticides on adrenal corticosterone formation, *Pestic. Biochem. Physiol.*, 1974, **4**, 254.
418. Angel, C., Starvation, stress and the blood-brain-barrier, *Dis. Nerv. Syst.*, 1969, **30**, 94.
419. Kling, T.G. and Long, K.R., Blood cholinesterase in previously stressed animals subjected to parathion, *J. Occup. Med.*, 1969, **11**, 82.

420. Baer,H., long term isolation stress and its effects on drug response in rodents, *Lab Animal Sci.*, 1971, **21**, 341.

421. Kesselring, J., Sewell, R.G., Gallus, J.A., Stiger, T.R. and Nearchou, N.I., Parachloroamphetamine toxicity in mice: Influence of body weights, sex and dose, *Pharmacol. Biochem. Behav.*, 1983, **18**, 821.

422. Gardocki, J.F., Schuler, M.E. and Goldstein, L., Reconsideration of the central nervous system pharmacology of amphetamine II Influence of pharmacologic agents on cumulative and total lethality in grouped and isolated mice, *Tox. Appl. Pharmacol.*, 1966, **9**, 536.

423. Weaver, L.C. and Kerley, T.L., Strain difference in response of mice to d-amphetamine, *J. Pharm. exptl. Ther.*, 1962, **135**, 240.

424. Spoerlein, M.T., Studies on acute morphine toxicity in grouped mice, *The Pharmacologist*, 1968, **10**, 172.

425. Balazs, T., Murphy, J.B. and Grice, H.C., The influence of environmental changes on the cardiotoxicity of isoprenaline in rats, *J. Pharm. Pharmacol.*, 1962, **14**, 750.

426. Yamauchi, C., Takahashi, H., Ando, A., Imaishi, N. and Nomura, T., Influence of environmental temperature on acute toxicity in laboratory mice (in Japanese), *Exp. Anim.*, 1967, **16**, 31.

427. Keplinger, M.L., Lanier, G.E. and Deichmann, W.B., Effects of environmental temperature on the acute toxicity of a number of compounds in rats, *Tox. Appl. Pharmacol.*, 1959, **1**, 156.

428. Selisko, O., Huntschel, G. and Ackermann, H., Über die Abhängijkeit der mittleren tödlichen dosis (LD_{50}) von exogenen Faktoren, *Arch. int. Pharmacodyn. Therap.*, 1963, **45**, 51.

429. Baetjer, A.M. and Smith, R., Effect of environmental temperature on reaction of mice to parathion, an anticholinesterase agent, *Am. J. Physiol.*, 1956, **186**, 39.

430. Ahdaya, S.M., Shah, P.V. and Guthrie, F.E., Thermoregulation in mice treated with parathion, carbaryl or DDT., *Tox. Appl. Pharmacol.*, 1978, **35**, 575.

431. Hovevey-Sion, D. and Kaplanski, J., Toxicity of digoxin in acutely and chronically heat-exposed rats, *Res. Comm. Chem. Path. Pharmacol.*, 1979, **25**, 517.

432. Zvi, Z.V. and Kaplanski, J., Effects of chronic heat exposure on drug metabolism in the rat, *J. Pharm. Pharmacol.*, 1980, **32**, 268.

433. Cremer, J.E. and Bligh, J., Body temperature and responses to drugs, *Br. Med. Bull.*, 1969, **25**, 299.

434. Cornwell, P.B. and Bull, J.O., Alphakill – a new rodenticide for mouse control, *Pest Control.*, 1967, **35**, 31.

435. Cornwell, P.B. Alphakill, A new rodenticide for mouse control, *Pharm. J.*, 1969, **202**, 74.

436. Snow, M.K. and Sheppard, M.J., Drug danger to domestic pets, *Vet. Rec.*, 1968, **82**, 553.

437. Usinger, W., Respiratorischer stoffwechsel und Korpertemperatur der weissen Maus in thermoindifferenter Umgebung, *Pflügers Archiv.*, 1957, **264**, 520.

438. Grigorowa, R. and Binnewies, S., Ueber die kombinierte wirkung von phosphoorganischen Pestiziden und erhoehter Umgebungstemparatur in, Inhalotorischen Kurzuersuchen an Ratten, i Toxikologische Aspekte, *Int. Arch. Arbeitsmed*, 1973, **31**, 295.

439. Boyd, C.E., Vinson, S.B. and Ferguson, D.E., Possible DDT resistance in two species of frogs, *Copeica No. 2*, 1963, **426**.

440. Kaplan, H.M. and Overpeck, J.G., Toxicity of halogenated hydrocarbon insecticides for the frog *Rana pipiens, Herpetologica*, 1964, **20**, 163.

441. Henderson, C., Pickering, Q.H. and Tarzwell, C.M., Relative toxicity of the chlorinated hydrocarbon insecticides to four species of fish, *Trans. Am. Fish Soc.*, 1959, **88**, 23.

442. Pickering, Q.H., Henderson, C. and Lemke, A.E., The Toxicity of organic phosphorus insecticides to different species of warm water fishes, *Trans. Am. Fish Soc.*, 1962, **81**, 175.

443. Schvartsman, S., Toxicology: Points of view of a tropical country in, *Proceedings of the 1st International Congress of Toxicology (Toronto, Canada)*. Academic Press – New York, San Francisco and London, 1978.

444. Smith, R.L. and Bababunine, E.A., Eds., *Toxicology in the Tropics*, Taylor and Francis Ltd., London, 1980.

445. Pimental, R. and Buckley, R.V., Influence of water hardness on fluoride toxicity to rainbow trout, *Environ. Tox. Chem.*, 1983, **2**, 381.

446. Lund, M., Resistance of rodents to rodenticides, *World Rev. Pest Control*, 1967, **6**, 131.

447. Ferguson, D.E., Culley, D.C., Cotton, W.D. and Dodds, R.P., Resistance to chlorinated hydrocarbon insecticides in three species of freshwater fish, *Bioscience*, 1964, **13**, 43.

448. Rowan, A.N., Alternatives to laboratory animals in, *Animals in Research*, Ed. Sperlinger, D., John Wiley and Sons Inc., 1981a.

449. Rowan, A.N., The LD_{50} test: A critique and suggestions for alternatives, *Pharm. Tech.*, 1981b, **5**, 64.

450. Rowan, A.N., *Of mice, models and men: A critique evaluation of animal research*, State University of New York Press, New York, 1984.

451. Godlovich, S., Godlovich, R. and Harris, J., *Animals men and models – An enquiry into the maltreatment of non-humans*, Victor Gallencz Ltd. London, 1971.

452. Clark, S.R.L., *The moral status of animals*, Clarendon Press, Oxford, 1977.

453. Rollin, B.E., *Animal rights and human morality*, Promethrics Books, New York, 1981.

454. Holden, C., New focus on replacing animals in the lab, *Science*, 1982, **215**, 35.

455. Dayan, A.D., Clark, B., Jackson, M., Morgan, H. and Charlesworth, F.A., Role of the LD_{50} test in the pharmaceutical industry, *The Lancet*, i, 1984, 555.

456. Krasovskii, G.N. and Ilnitskii, A.P., The question of the use of tissue culture methods in sanitary and toxicological studies, (in Russian), *Gig. Sanit.*, 1967, **32**, 66.

457. Dawson, M., Three R's of animal experimentation: Reduction, replacement and refinement, *Pharm. J.*, 1984, **232**, 607.

458. Dawson, M., *In vitro* systems in basic biometrical research in, *The Future of Animals, Cells, Models and Systems in Research, Development, Education and Testing*, (Proceedings of a Symposium – No Editor), National Academy of Sciences, Washington DC, 1977.

459. Balls, M. and Rao, R., Organ culture in pharmacology in, *The Use of Alternatives in Drug Research*. Eds., Rowan, A.N. and Stratmann, C.J., Macmillan Press Ltd., 1980.

460. Nardone, R.M., Tissue culture systems in toxicity testing in, *The Use of Alternatives in Drug Research*, Eds., Rowan, A.N. and Stratmann, C.J., Macmillan Press Ltd., 1980.

461. Paine, A.J., Ord, M.J., Neal, G.E. and Skilliter, D.N., Cell models in the study of toxic mechanisms in, *The Use of Alternatives in Drug Research*, Eds., Rowan, A.N. and Stratmann, C.J., Macmillan Press Ltd., 1980.

462. Rees, K.R., Cells in culture in toxicity testing: A review, *J. Roy. Soc. Med.*, 1980, **73**, 261.

463. Stammati, A.P., Silano, V. and Zucco, F., Toxicology investigations with cell culture systems, *Toxicology*, 1981, **20**, 91.

464. Ekwall, B., Screening of toxic compounds in tissue culture, *Toxicology*, 1980, **17**, 127.

465. Ekwall, B., Correlation between cytotoxicity *in vitro*, and LD_{50} values. *Acta. Pharmacol. Toxicol.*, 1983, **52**, Supp. II, 80.

466. Elizarova, O.N. and Nuzhdina, D.P., Application of tissue culture for determining the toxicity of pesticides (in English), *Gig. Sanit.*, 1971, **36**, 83.

467. Dillingham, E.O., Mast, R.W., Bass, G.E. and Autian, J., Toxicity of methyl- and halogen-substituted alcohol in tissue culture relative to structure-activity models and acute toxicity in mice, *J. Pharm. Sci.*, 1973, **62**, 22.

468. Walum, E. and Peterson, A., Acute toxicity testing in culture of mouse neuroblastoma cells, *Acta Pharmacol. Toxicol.*, 1983, **52**, Supp. II, 100.

469. Balls, M.N. and Clothier, R., Differential cell and organ culture in toxicity testing, *Acta Pharmacol. Toxicol.*, 1983, **52**, Supp. II, 115.

470. Nebert, D.W., Genetic and environmental factors influencing drug metabolism in, *Perinatal Pharmacology: Problems and Priorities*, Eds., Davies, J. and Hwang, J.C., Raven Pree, New York.

471. Jnutson, J.C. and Poland, A., 2,3,7,8-Tetrachlorodibenzo-*p*-dioxin: Failure to demonstrate toxicity in twenty-three cultured cell types, *Tox. Appl. Pharmacol.*, 1980, **54**, 377.

472. Smith, C.G., Grady, J.E. and Northam, J.I., Relationship between cytotoxicity *in vitro* and whole animal toxicity, *Cancer Chemotherap. Reps.*, 1963, No. 30, 9.

473. Heilbronn, E., Methods using tissue preparations and isolated biomolecules, *Acta Pharmacol. Toxicol.*, 1983, **52**, Supp. II, 138.

474. Nardone, R., The LD_{50} test and *in vitro* toxicology strategies, *Acta Pharmacol. Toxicol.*, 1983, **52**, Supp. II, 65.

475. Geothals, F., Krack, G., Deboyser, D., Vossen, P. and Roberfroid, M., Critical biochemical functions of isolated hepatocytes as sensitive indicators of chemical toxicity, *Fund. Appl. Toxicol.*, 1984, **4**, 441.

476. Robison, W.H., Acute toxicity of sodium monofluoroacetate to cattle, *J. Wildlife Mgt.*, 1970, **34**, 647.

477. Atzert, S.P., A review of sodium monofluoroacetate (compound 1080) – its properties, toxicology and use in predator and rodent control, *US Fish Wildl. Serv. Spoc. Sci. Rep. Wildl. No. 146*, 1971.

478. Peters, R.A., *Biochemical Lesions and Lethal Synthesis*, Pergamon Press, 1963.

479. Mager, P.D. and Geege, A., Quantitative struktor-toxizitats-bezichungen bei phosphorsänreestern (in German), *Pharmazie*, 1980, **35**, 806.

480. O'Brien, R.D., Kinetics of the carbamorylation of cholinesterase, *Mol. Pharmacol.*, 1968, **4**, 121.

481. Ellin, R.I. and Wills, J.H., Oximes antagonistic to inhibitors of cholinesterase (Part 1), *J. Pharm. Sci.*, 1964, **53**, 995.

482. Ellin, R.I. and Wills, J.H., Oximes antagonistic to inhibitors of cholinesterase (Part 2), *J. Pharm. Sci.*, 1964, **53**, 1143.

483. Ashani, Y. and Cohen, S., Structure-activity relationship of some new reactivators of phosphorylated cholinesterase, *Israel J. Chem.*, 1965, **3**, 116.

484. Pickering, C.E. and Pickering, R.G., Methods for the estimation of acetylcholinesterase activity in the plasma and brain of laboratory animals given carbamates or organophosphorus compounds, *Arch. Toxicol.*, 1971, **27**, 292.

485. Pickering, R.G. and Pickering, C.E., Methods for the estimation of acetylcholinesterase activity in the erythrocytes of laboratory animals given

carbamates or organophosphate compounds, *Arch. Toxicol.*, 1974, **31**, 197.

486. Andersen, R.A., Gargas, I., Gaare, G. and Fonnum, F., Inhibition of acetyl-cholinesterase from different species by organophosphorus compounds, carbamates and methylsulphorylfluoride, *Gen. Pharmac.*, 1977, **8**, 331.

487. Lovell, J.B., The relationship of anticholinesterase activity, penetration and insect and mammalian toxicity of certain organophosphorus insecticides, *J. Econ. Entomol.*, 1963, **56**, 310.

488. Cheymol, J., Chabrier, P., Thuong, N.T., Rioult, P. and Goyer, R., Contribution a l'etude chronique et pharmacologique des derivies de l'acide orthophosphorique (in French), *Med. Pharmacol. exp.*, 1966, **14**, 305.

489. Whitehouse, L.W. and Ecobichon, D.J., Paraoxinformation and hydrolysis by mammalian liver, *Pestic. Biochem.*, 1975, **5**, 314.

490. Litterst, C.L., Mimnaugh, E.G., Reagan, R.L. and Gram, T.E., Comparison of *in vitro* drug metabolism by lung, liver and kidney of several common laboratory species, *Drug Metab. Dispos.*, 1975, **3**, 259.

491. Youdim, M.B.H. and Paykel, E.S., Eds., *Monoamine Oxidase Inhibitors – the State of the Art*, John Wiley and Sons, Ltd., 1981.

492. Ridgeway, L.P. and Karnofsky, D.A., The effects of metals on the chick embryo: Toxicity and production of abnormalities in development, *Ann. N.Y. Acad. Sci.*, 1952, **55**, 203.

493. McLaughlin, J. Jr., and Mutchler, M.K., Toxicity of some chemicals measured by injection into chicken eggs, *Fed. Proc.*, 1962, **21**, 450.

494. Hemminki, K., Toxicity of rubber chemicals in the chicken embryo: How to interpret results from animal tests, *Scan. J. Work environ. Hlth.*, 1983, **9**, Supp. 2, 73.

495. Korhonen, A., Hemminki, K. and Vainio, H., Toxicity of rubber chemicals towards three-day chicken embryos, *Scan. J. Work. environ. Hlth.*, 1983, **9**, 115.

496. Walker, N.E., Distribution of chemicals injected into fertile eggs and its effect upon apparent toxicity, *Tox. Appl. Pharmacol.*, 1967, **10**, 290.

497. Vesely, D., Vesela, D. and Jelinek, R., Nineteen mycotoxins tested on chicken embryos, *Tox. Letters*, 1982, **13**, 239.

498. Khera, K.S. and Lyon, D.A., Chick and duck embryos in the evaluation of pesticide toxicity, *Tox. Appl. Pharmacol.*, 1968, **13**, 1.

499. Gibaldi, M. and Grundhsfer, B., Drug transport: VI Functional integrity of rat everted small intestine with respect of passive transfer, *J. Pharm. Sci.*, 1972, **61**, 116.

500. Dolvisio, J.T., Billups, J.V., Dittert, L.W., Sugita, E.T. and Swintosky, J.V., Drug absorption: I An *in situ* rat gut technique yielding realistic absorption rates, *J. Pharm. Sci.*, 1969, **58**, 1196.

501. Pekas, J.C., Uptake and transport of pesticidal carbamates by evented sacs of rat small intestine, *Canad. J. Physiol. Pharmacol.*, 1971a, **49**, 14.

502. Pekas, J.C., Intestinal metabolism and transport of naphthyl *N*-methyl carbamate *in vitro* (rats), *Amer. J. Physiol.*, 1971b, **220**, 2009.

503. Houston, J.B., Upshall, D.G. and Bridges, J.W., A re-evaluation of the importance of partition coefficient in the gastrointestinal absorption of nutrients, *J. Pharmacol. exptl. Ther.*, 1974, **189**, 244.

504. Houston, J.B., Upshall, D.G. and Bridges, J.W., Further studies using carbamate esters on model compounds to investigate the role of lipophilicity in the gastrointestinal absorption of foreign compounds, *J. Pharmacol. exptl. Ther.*, 1975, **195**, 67.

505. Levine, R.R., McNary, W.F., Kornguth, P.J. and LeBlanc, R., Histological

re-evaluation of everted gut technique for studying intestinal absorption, *Eur. J. Pharmacol.*, 1970, **9**, 211.

506. Michaels, A.S., Chandrasekaran, S.K. and Shaw, J.E., Drug permeation through human skin: Theory and *in vitro* experimental measurement, *A.I.Ch.E.*, 1975, **21**, 985.

507. Cooper, E.R., Pharmacokinetics of skin penetration, *J. Pharm. Sci.*, 1976, **65**, 1396.

508. Chandrasekaran, S.K., Bayne, W. and Shaw, J.E., Pharmacokinetics of drug permeation through human skin, *J. Pharm. Sci.*, 1978, **67**, 1370.

509. Dyer, A., Hayes, G.G., Wilson, J.G. and Catterall, R., Diffusion through skin and model systems, *Int. J. Cosmetic. Sci.*, 1979, **1**, 91.

510. Kubota, K. and Ishizaki, T., A theoretical consideration of percutaneous drug absorption. *J. Pharmacokin. Biopharm.*, 1985, **13**, 55.

511. Mehendale, H.M., Angevine, L.S. and Ohmiya, Y., The isolated perfused lung: A critical evaluation, *Toxicology*, 1981, **21**, 1.

512. Kenega, E.E., Test-organisms and methods useful for early assessment of acute toxicity of chemicals, *Environ. Sci. Technol.*, 1978, **12**, 1322.

513. Kaiser, H.E., *Species-specific potential of invertebrates for toxicological research*, University Park Press, Baltimore, 1980.

514. Ord, M.J., A cell system for use in toxicology studies, *ATLA*, 1981, **9**, 7.

515. Sovak, M., Ranganathan, R. and Mutzell, W., Determination of lethal dose in a protozoa: Screening of contrast media toxicity, *Invest. Radiol.*, 1981, **16**, 438.

516. Kordan, H., Responses of whole plant systems to pharmacological agents, *ATLA*, 1981, **9**, 24.

517. Craig, P.N. and Enslein, K., Structure-activity in hazard assessment in *Hazard Assessment of Chemicals – Current Developments*, Eds., Saxena, J. and Fisher, F., Academic Press, New York, 1981.

518. Tute, M.S., Mathematical Modelling in, *Animals and Alternatives in Toxicology*, Eds., Balls, M., Riddell, R.J. and Worden, A.N., Academic Press, London, 1983.

519. Golberg, L., Ed., Structure activity correlation as a predictive tool in, *Toxicology: Fundamentals, Methods and Applications*, Hemisphere Publishing Corp., 1983.

520. Martin, Y.C., Studies of relationships between structural properties and biological activity by Hansch Analysis in, *Structure–activity Correlation as a Predictive Tool in Toxicology*, Ed., Golberg, L., Hemisphere Publishing Corp., 1983, 77.

521. Martin, Y.C., A practitioner's perspective of the role of quantitative structure–activity analysis in medical chemistry, *J. Med. Chem.*, 1981, **24**, 229.

522. Martin, Y.C., The quantitative relationships between pK_a, ionization and drug potency in, *Physical Chemical Properties of Drugs*, Eds., Yalowsky, S., Sinkula, A. and Valvani, S.C., Marcel-Dekker, New York, 1980.

523. Jurs, P.C., Studies of relationships between molecular structure and biological activity by pattern recognition methods in, *Structure–activity Correlation as a Predictive Tool in Toxicology*, Ed., Golberg, L., Hemisphere Publishing Corp., 1983, 93.

524. Wipke, W.T., Ouchi, G.I. and Chou, J.T., Computer assisted prediction of metabolism in, *Structure–activity Correlations as a Predictive Tool in Toxicology*, Ed., Golberg, L., Hemisphere Publishing Corp., 1983, 151.

525. Chignell, C.E., Overview of molecular parameters that relate to biological activity in toxicology in *Structure–activity Correlation as a Predictive Tool in Toxicology*, Ed., Golberg., Hemisphere Publishing Corp., 1983, 61.

526. Purcell, W.P., Bass, G.E. and Clayton, J.M., *Strategy of Drug Design: A Guide to Biological Activity*, John Wiley and Sons, 1973.
527. Ferguson, J., The use of chemical potentials as indices of toxicity, *Proc. Roy. Soc. Series B*, 1939, **127**, 387.
528. Brodie, B.B. and Hogben, C.A.M., Some physico–chemical factors in drug action, *J. Pharm. Pharmacol.*, 1957, **9**, 345.
529. Albert, A., *Selective Toxicity*, Chapman and Hall, London (7th Edition), 1985.
530. McGowan, J.C., Partition coefficients and biological activities, *Nature*, 1963, **200** 1317.
531. Glave, W.R. and Hansch, C., Relationship between lipophilic character and anaesthetic activity, *J. Pharm. Sci.*, 1972, **61**, 589.
532. Lien, E.J. and Tong, G.L., Physiochemical properties and percutaneous absorption of drugs, *J. Soc. Cosmet. Chem.*, 1973, **24**, 371.
533. Durden, J.A., Jr., Acute oral toxicity of 2-alkyl and 2,6-dialkylanilenes: Correlation with liphophilicity, *J. Med. Chem.*, 1973, **16**, 1316.
534. Chiou, C.T., Freed, V.H., Schmedding, D.W. and Kohnert, R.L., Partition coefficient and bioaccumulation of selected organic chemicals, *Environ. Sci. Technol.*, 1977, **11**, 475.
535. Leo, A., Hansch, C. and Elkins, D., Partition coefficient and their uses, *Chem. Rev.*, 1971, **71**, 525.
536. Penniston, J.T., Beckett, L., Bentley, D.C. and Hansch, C., Passive permeation of organic compounds through biological tissue: A non-steady state theory, *Mol. Pharmacol.*, 1969, **5**, 333.
537. Khalil, S. and Martin, A., Drug transport through model membranes and its correlation with solubility parameters, *J. Pharm. Sci.*, 1967, **56**, 1225.
538. Birge, W.J. and Cassidy, R.A., Structure–activity relationships in aquatic toxicology, *Fund. Appl. Toxicol.*, 1983, **3**, 359.
539. Zahradnik, R., Correlation of the biological activity of organic compounds by means of the linear free-energy relationship, *Experientia*, 1962, **18**, 534.
540. Lukovits, I., Quantitative structure–activity relationships employing independent quantum chemical indices, *J. Med. Chem.*, 1983, **26**, 1104.
541. Tanii, H. and Hashimoto, K., Structure–toxicity relationship of acrylates and methacrylates, *Toxicology Letters*, 1982, **11**, 125.
542. Bowden, K. and Coombs, T.J., Quantitative structure–activity relationships in, *Progress in Pharmaceutical Research*, SCI Critical Reports on Applied Chemistry, Vol. 4, Blackwell Scientific Publications, 1982.
543. Seydel, J.K. and Schaefer, K-J., Quantitative structure–pharmacokinetic relationship and drug design, *Pharmac. Ther.*, 1982, **15**, 131.
544. Dunn III, W.J. and Wold, S., Relationships between chemical structure and biological activity modelled by SIMCA pattern recognition, *Bioorganic Chemistry*, 1980, **9**, 505.
545. Richards, W.G., *Quantum Pharmacology*, Butterworths, 1977.
546. Autian, J., Structure–toxicity relationships of acrylic monomers, *Environ. Hlth. Perspect.*, 1975, **11**, 141.
547. Hansch, C., Quantitative approaches to pharmacological structure–activity relationships in, *International Encyclopaedia of Pharmacology and Therapeutics*, Ed., Cavallito, C.J., Pergamon Press, Oxford, 1973.
548. Lawrence, W.H., Bass, G.E., Purcell, W.P. and Autian, J., Use of mathematical models in the study of structure–activity relationships of dental compounds: 1. Esters of acrylic and methacrylic acids, *J. Dental Res.*, 1972, **51**, 526.
549. Lyublina, E.I. and Rabotnikova, L.V., The possibility of predetermining the toxicities of volatile organic compounds from their physical constants (in Russian). *Hyg. i Sanit.*, 1971, **36**, 23.

550. Tute, M.S., Principles and practice of Hansch Analysis: A guide to structure–activity correlation for the medicinal chemist in, *Advances in Drug Research*, Vol. VI, Eds., Harper, N.J. and Simmonds, A.B., Academic Press, 1971.

551. Kier, L.B., *Molecular Orbital Theory in Drug Research*, Academic Press, 1971.

552. Brakhnova, I.T. and Samsonov, G.V., The dependence of the toxicity of some chemical substances on their electronic structure (in Russian), *Poroshkovaya Metallurgiya*, 1966, **6**, 101.

553. Bawden, D., Structure–toxicity studies in, *Animals and Alternatives in Toxicology*, Eds., Balls, M., Riddell, R.J. and Worden, A.N., Academic Press, 1983.

554. Carson, E.R., Mathematical models in pharmacotoxity in, *Animals and Alternatives in Toxicology*, Eds., Balls, M., Riddell, R.J. and Worden, A.N., Academic Press, 1983.

555. Dearden, J.C., Quantitative use of structural designs in, *Animals and Alternatives in Toxicology*, Eds., Balls, M., Riddell, R.J. and Worden, A.N., Academic Press, 1983.

556. Frankie, R., Oehme, P. and Barth, A., Mathematical model of dose–activity relationships, *Environmental Quality and Safety*, 1975, **3**, (Suppl.), 461.

557. Elliott, J.R., Use of regression diagnostics in QSAR studies, *Biometrics*, 1983, **39**, 804.

558. Daniels, K.L., Goyert, J.C., Strand, D.H. and Farrell, M.P., Statistical analysis of structure–activity relationships, *Fund. Appl. Toxicol.*, 1983, **3**, 350.

559. Wold, S., Herllberg, S. and Dunn III, W.J., Complete methods for the assessment of acute toxicity, *Acta Pharmacol. Toxicol.*, 1983, **52**, (Suppl. II.), 158.

560. Luecke, R.H., Thomason, L.E. and Wosilait, W.D., Physiological flow model for drug elimination interactions in the rat, *Computer Programs in Biomedicine*, 1980, **11**, 88.

561. Tuey, D.B. and Matthews, H.B., Use of a physiological compartmental model for the rat to describe the pharmacokinetics of several chlorinated biphenyls in the mouse, *Drug Metab. Dispos.*, 1980, **8**, 397.

562. Eschenroeder, A., Irvine, E., Lloyd, A., Tashima, C. and Tran, K., Computer simulation models for assessment of toxic substances in, *Dynamics, Exposure and Hazard Assessment of Toxic Chemicals*, Ed., Haque, R., Ann Arbor Science Publishers Inc., Ann Arbor, 1980.

563. Colburn, W.A., Simultaneous pharmacokinetic and pharmacodynamic modelling, *J. Pharmacokin. Biopharm.*, 1981, **9**, 367.

564. Metzler, C.M. and Tong, D.D.M., Computational problems of computer models with Mickaelis–Menten-type elimination, *J. Pharm. Sci.*, 1981, **70**, 733.

565. Yamamoto, W.S. and Walton, E.S., On the evaluation of the physiological model, *Ann. Rev. Biophys., Bioeng.*, 1975, **4**, 81.

566. Adamson, G.W., Bawden, D. and Saggers, D.T., Quantitative structure–activity relationship studies of acute toxicity (LD_{50}) in a large series of herbicidal benzimidazoles, *Pestic. Sci.*, 1984, **15**, 31.

567. Enselein, K., Lander, T.R., Tomb, M.E. and Craig, P.N., *A Predictive Model for estimating Rat Oral LD_{50} Values*, Princeton Scientific Publishers Inc., Princeton N.J., 1983.

568. Rekker, R.F., LD_{50} values: Are they about to become predictable?, *TIPS*, 1980, (October issue), 383.

569. Tattersall, M.L., Statistics and the LD_{50} study, *Arch. Toxicol.*, 1982, **51**, (Suppl. 5), 267.

570. Bass, R., Günzel, P., Henschler, D., König, J., Lorke, D., Neubert, D., Schütz, E., Schuppan, D. and Zbinden, G., LD_{50} versus acute toxicity, *Arch. Toxicol.*, 1982, **51**, 183.

571. Überla, K. and Schneiders, B., In reference to the paper by Bass *et al* (Letter to the Editor), *Arch. Toxicol.*, 1982, **51**, 187.

572. British Toxicological Society (Working Party on Toxicity), A new approach to the classification of substances and preparations on the basis of their acute toxicity, *Human Toxicol.*, 1984, **3**, 85.

573. Winne, D., Zur plannung von versuchen: Wieviel versuchseinheiten? *Arzneim. - Forsch.*, 1968, **18**, 1611.

574. Brown, V.K., The LD_{50} value – a frequently missapplied concept, *ATLA*, 1984, **12**, 75.

575. Majda, A., Optimalisation endeavour of the numerousness of animals in experimental groups in acute toxicity routine estimation assays on rats, *Zwierzete Lab.*, 1976, **13**, 37.

576. Weil, C.S., Carpenter, C.P., West, J.S. and Smyth, H.F., Jr., Reproducibility of single oral dose toxicity testing, *Am. Industr. Hyg. J.*, 1966, **27**, 483.

577. Weil, C.S. and Wright, G.J., Intra- and interlaboratory comparative evaluation of single oral test, *Tox. Appl. Pharmacol.*, 1967, **11**, 378.

578. Peacock, D.B. and Palmateer, S.C., Comparison of EPA animal biological laboratory and company laboratory efficacy data for Federally registered rat and mouse baits in, *Vertebrate Pest Control and Management Material (ASTM STP 680)*, Ed., Beck, J.R., American Society for Testing and Materials, Philadelphia, 1979.

579. Griffith, J.F., Interlaboratory variations in the determination of acute oral LD_{50}, *Tox. Appl. Pharmacol.*, 1964, **6**, 726.

580. Allmark, M.G., A collaborative study on the acute toxicity of several drugs, *J. Am. Pharm. Assoc.*, 1951, **40**, 27.

581. Hunter, W.J., Lingk, W. and Recht, P., Intercomparison study on the determination of single administration toxicity in rats, *J. Assoc. Off. Anal. Chem.*, 1979, **62**, 864.

582. Lebeau, J.E., The role of the LD_{50} determination in drug safety evaluation, *Reg. Tox. Pharmacol.*, 1983, **3**, 71.

583. Cliff, K.S., Agriculture – The occupation hazards, *Public Hlth. Lond.*, 1981, **95**, 15.

584. Copplestone, J.F., A global view of pesticide safety in, *Pesticide Management and Insecticide Resistance*, Eds., Watson, D.L. and Brown, A.W.A., Academic Press, 1977.

585. Bull, D., *A Growing Problem: Pesticides in the Third World Poor*, Oxfam, Oxford, 1982.

586. Rowe, W.D., *An Anatomy of Risk*, John Wiley and Sons, 1977.

587. Crossland, J. and Shea, K.P., The hazards of impurities, *Environment*, 1983, **15**, 35.

588. Implementing the Seveso Directive: Report of a conference held in London (October 1983), Oyez Scientific and Technical Services Ltd., London.

589. Report on 2,4,5-T – A report of the panel on herbicides of the President's Science Advisory Committee, Executive Office of the President of the USA, 1971.

590. Umetsu, N., Grose, F.H., Allahyari, R., Abu-el-Haj, S. and Fukuto, T.R., Effect of impurities on the mammalian toxicity of technical malathion and acephate, *J. Agric. Food Chem.*, 1977, **25**, 946.

591. Baker, E.L., Jr., Zack, M., Miles, J.W., Alderman, L., Warren, M., Dobbin, R.D., Miller, S. and Teeters, W.R., Epidemic malathion poisoning in Pakistan malaria workers, *The Lancet*, i, 1978, 31.

592. Bellet, E.M. and Casida, J.E., Bicylic phosphorus esters: High toxicity without cholinesterase inhibition, *Science*, 1973, **182**, 1135.

593. Hilado, C.J. and Cumming, H.J., Short-term LD_{50} values: An update on available information, *Fire Technology*, 1978, **14**, 46.

594. Weger, N.P., Treatment of cyanide poisoning with 4-dimethyl-aminophenol (DMAP) – Experimental and clinical overview, *Fund. Appl. Toxicol.*, 1983, **3**, 387.

595. DiCarlo, F.J., Seifter, J. and DeCarlo, V.J., Assessment of the hazards of poly-brominated biphenyls, *Environ. Hlth. Perspect.*, 1978, **23**, 351.

596. Simpson, L.L., The origin, structure and pharmacological activity of Botulinum toxin, *Pharmacol. Revs.*, 1981, **33**, 155.

597. Hails, M.R. and Crane, T.D., Plant poisoning in animals: A bibliography from the World Literature 1960–1979, *Vet. Bull.*, 1982, **52**, Pt 1, 557; Pt 2, 679: Pt 3, 783; Pt 4, 895; Pt 5, 1023.

598. Kingshorn, A.D., Ed., *Toxic Plants.*, Columbia University Press, New York, 1979.

599. Bower, D.J., Hart, R.J., Matthews, P.A. and Howden, M.E.H., Non-protein neurotoxins, *Clin. Toxicol.*, 1981, **18**, 813.

600. Karlsson, E., Chemistry of some potent animal toxins, *Experienta*, 1973, **29**, 1319.

601. Mebs, D., Chemistry of animal venoms, poisons and toxins, *Experienta*, 1973, **29**, 1328.

602. Kao, C.Y., Tetrodotoxin, saxitoxin and their significance in the study of excitation phenomena, *Pharmacol. Revs.*, 1966, **18**, 997.

603. Clark, B. and Smith, D.A., Pharmacokinetics and toxicity testing, *CRC Critical Revs. Toxicol.*, 1984, **12**, 343.

604. Mikheev, M., Toxicity prediction in association with evaluation and risk assessment of chemicals in, *Health Aspects of Chemical Safety (Interim Document No. 6): Risk Assessment*, World Health Organisation, Regional Office for Europe, Copenhagen.

605. Lorke, D., A new approach to practical acute toxicity testing, *Arch. Toxicol.*, 1983, **54**, 275.

606. Müller, H. and Kley, H-P., Retrospective study on the reliability of an 'approximate LD_{50}' determined with a small number of animals, *Arch. Toxicol.*, 1982, **51**, 189.

607. Schütz, E. and Fuchs, H., A new approach to minimizing the number of animals used in acute toxicity testing and optimizing the information of test results, *Arch. Toxicol.*, 1982, **51**, 197.

608. Benson, W.W., The pesticide fire; a potential killer, *Fire Command*, 1973, (February issue), 1.

609. Schantz, E.J. and Sugiyama, H., The toxins of *Clostridium botulinum* in *Essays in Toxicology*, Vol. 5, Eds., Hayes, W.J., Jr., Academic Press, 1971.

610. Refshauge, W., The place for international standards in conducting research on humans, *Bull. Wld Hlth Org.*, 1977, 55 (Suppl. 2), 133.

611. Weiner, J.S., The ethics of human experimentation in, *The Principles and Practice of Human Physiology*, Eds., Edholm, O.G. and Weiner, J.S., Academic Press, 1975.

612. National Academy of Sciences (Washington DC), Experiments and research with humans; Values in conflict. Academy Forum (3rd of Series), 1975.

613. Hume, C.W., The strategy and tactics of experimentation, *The Lancet*, 1957, **273**, 1049.

614. World Health Organization; Recommended classification of pesticides by hazard, *WHO Chronicle*, 1957, **29**, 397.

615. Finney, D.J., The median lethal dose and its estimation, *Arch. Toxicol.*, 1985, **56**, 215.

616. Debanne, S.M. and Haller, H.S., Evaluation of statistical methodologies for estimation of median effective dose, *Tox. Appl. Pharmacol.*, 1985, **79**, 274.

617. Waud, D.R. and Waud, B.E., Heuristic and practical graphing of dose–response relationships, *TIPS*, 1985, **6**, 26.
618. King, L.A., Ferguson's Principle and the prediction of fatal drug levels in blood, *Human Toxicol.*, 1985, **4**, 273.
619. Hudson, S.A., Drug administration and food, *Pharmacy Update.*, 1985, **1**, 337.
620. Dashiell, O.L. and Kennedy, Jr., G.L., The effects of fasting on the acute oral toxicity of nine chemicals in the rat, *J. Appl. Toxicol.*, 1984, **4**, 320.
621. Atterwill, C.K. and Steele, C.E., (Eds.), *In Vitro Methods In Toxicology*, Cambridge University Press, Cambridge, 1988.
622. Debanne, S.M. and Haller, H.S., Evaluation of statistical methodologies for estimation of median effective dose, *Tox. Appl. Pharmacol.*, 1985, **79**, 274.
623. Bowser, P.A., White, R.J. and Nugteren, D.H., Location and nature of the epidermal permeability barrier, *Int. J. Cosmet. Sci.*, 1986, **8**, 125.
624. Szakall, A., Hautphysiologische Forschung und Gesunderhaltung der Haut, *Fette und Seifen*, 1951, **53**, 399.
625. Allen, R.E., Thoshinky, M.J., Stallone, R.J. and Hunt, T.K., Corrosive injuries of the stomach, *Arch. Surg.*, 1970, **100**, 409.
626. Sereni, F. and Principi, N., Developmental Toxicology, *Ann. Revs Pharmacol.*, 1968, **8**, 453.
627. Mirkin, B.L., Developmental Pharmacology, *Ann. Revs Pharmacol.*, 1970, **10**, 255.
628. Yaffe, S.J. and Juchau, M.R., Perinatal Toxicology, *Ann. Revs Pharmacol.*, 1974, **14**, 219.
629. Baker, S.R. and Rogul, M. (Eds), *Environmental Toxicology and the Aging Processes.*, [Progress in Clinical and Biological Research, Volume 228], Alan R. Liss, Inc., New York, 1987.
630. Miners, J.O., Robson, R.A. and Birkett, D.J., Paracetamol metabolism in pregnancy, *Brit. J. Clin. Pharm.*, 1986, **22**, 359.
631. Kalow, W., Goedde, H.W. and Agarwal, D.P., (Eds), *Ethnic Differences in Reactions to Drugs and Xenobiotics*, [Progress in Clinical and Biological Research, Volume 214], Alan R. Liss, Inc., New York, 1986.
632. Abrams, J., Nitrate Delivery Systems, In *Modern Concepts in Nitrate Delivery Systems.*, (Eds) A.A.J. Goldberg and D.G. Parsons, *Royal Society of Medicine International Congress and Symposium Series No. 54*, Academic Press, London and Royal Society of Medicine, London, 1983.
633. Campbell, K.I., Inhalation toxicology, *Clin. Toxicol.*, 1976, **9**, 849.
634. Witschi, H. and Nettesheim, P., (Eds), *Mechanisms in Respiratory Toxicology (Volumes 1 & 2)*, C.R.C. Press, Inc., Boca Raton, Fa., 1982.
635. Phalen, R.F., Mannix, R.C. and Drew, R.T., Inhalation exposure methodology, *Environ. Hlth Perspect.*, 1984, **56**, 23.
636. Miller, R.R., Letts, R.L., Potts, W.J. and McKenna, M.J., Improved methodology for generating controlled test atmospheres, *Am. industr. Hyg. Ass. J.*, 1980, **41**, 844.
637. Sabourin, P.J., Chen, B.T., Lucifer, G., Birnbaum, L.S., Fisher, E. and Henderson, R.F., Effect of dose on the absorption and excretion of (^{14}C) benzene administered orally or be inhalation in rats and mice, *Tox. Appl. Pharmacol.*, 1987, **87**, 325.
638. Silcock, S.R., Refinement of experimental procedures, *ATLA*, 1986, **14**, 72.
639. Piek, T. (Ed.), *Venoms of the Hymenoptera*, Academic Press, 1986.
640. Klonne, D.R., Ulrich, C.E., Weissmann, J. and Morgan, A.K., Acute inhalation toxicity of aliphatic (C_1 – C_5) nitrites in rats, *Fundam. Appl. Toxicol.*, 1987, **8**, 101.
641. Sloan, K.B., Koch, S.A.M., Silver, K.G. and Flowers, F.P., Use of solubility

parameters of drug and vehicle to predict flux through skin, *J. Invest. Dermatol.*, 1986, **87**, 244.

642. Meier, J. and Theakston, R.D.G., Approximate LD_{50} determinations of snake venoms using eight to ten experimental animals, *Toxicon*, 1986, **24**, 395.

643. Vale, J.A., Meredith, T.J. and Proudfoot, A.T., Syrup of ipecacuahna: Is it really useful? *Brit. Med. J.*, 1986, **293**, 1321.

644. Poland, A. and Kimbrough, R.D., (Eds), *Biological Mechanisms of Dioxin Action*, Banbury Report No. 18, Cold Spring Harbor Laboratory, 1984.

645. Fraser, N.C., Accidental poisoning deaths in British children, 1958–1977, *Brit. Med. J.*, 1980, **280**, 1595.

646. Saddique, A. and Peterson, C.D., Thallium poisoning; A review, *Vet. Hum. Toxicol.*, 1983, **25**, 116.

647. Woodhouse, K.W. and Wynne, H., The pharmacokinetics of non-steroidal anti-inflammatory drugs in the elderly, *Clin. Pharmacokin.*, 1987, **12**, 111.

648. Schmidt–Nielsen, K., Energy metabolism, body size and problems of scaling, *Fed. Proc.*, 1970, **29**, 1524.

649. Weiss, M., Sziegoleit, W. and Forster, W., Dependence of pharmacokinetic parameters on the body weight, *Int. J. Clin. Pharm. Ther. Toxicol.*, 1977, **15**, 572.

650. Davidson, I.W.F., Parker, J.C. and Beliles, R.P., Biological basis for extrapolation across mammalian species, *Reg. Toxicol. Pharmacol.*, 1986, **6**, 211.

651. Sigell, L.T., Kapp, F.T., Fusaro, G.A., Nelson, E.D. and Falck, R.S., Popping and snorting volatile nitrites: a current fad for getting high, *Amer. J. Psychiatr.*, 1978, **135**, 1216.

652. Watson, J.M., *Solvent Abuse; the Adolescent Epidemic?*, Croom Helm, London, 1986.

653. Giovacchini, R.P., Abusing the volatile organic chemicals, *Reg. Toxicol. Pharmacol.*, 1985, **5**, 18.

654. Beliles, R.P., The influence of pregnancy on the acute toxicity of compounds in mice, *Tox. Appl. Pharmacol.*, 1972, **23**, 537.

655. Brownlee, K.A., Hodges, J.L. and Rosenblatt, M., The up-and-down method with small samples., *J. Amer. Statist. Ass.*, 1953, **48**, 262.

656. Wetherill, G.B., Sequential estimation of quantal response curves, *J. Roy. Statist. Soc. [B]*, 1963, **25**, 1.

657. Choi, S.C., An investigation of Wetherill's method of estimation for the up-and-down experiment, *Biometrics.*, 1971, **27**, 961.

658. Dixon, W.J., The up-and-down method for small samples, *J. Amer. Statis. Ass.*, 1965, **60**, 967.

659. Hsi, B.P., The multiple sample up-and-down method in bioassay, *J. Amer. Statist. Ass.*, 1969, **64**, 147.

660. Bruce, R.D., An up-and-down procedure for acute toxicity testing, *Fundam. Appl. Toxicol.*, 1985, **5**, 151.

661. Bruce, R.D., A confirmatory study of the up-and-down method for acute oral toxicity testing, *Fundam. Appl. Toxicol.*, 1987, **8**, 97.

662. Anon., Thallium poisoning in Guyana; a national crisis, *The Lancet*, i, 1987, 604.

663. O'Flaherty, E.J., Dose dependent toxicity, *Comments on Toxicology.*, 1986, **1**, 23.

664. Morris, J.B., Clay, R.J. and Cavanagh, D.G., Species differences in upper respiratory tract deposition of acetone and ethanol vapors *Fundam. Appl. Toxicol.*, 1986, **7**, 671.

665. Renwick, A.G., Pharmacokinetics in Toxicology in, *Principles and Methods of Toxicology*, (Ed. A.W. Hayes), Raven Press, New York, 1982.

666. Bonati, M. Jiritano, L., Bortolotti, A., Gaspari, F., Fillippeschi, S., Puidgemont,

A and Garattini, S., Caffeine distribution in acute toxic response among inbred mice, *Tox. Lett.*, 1985, **29**, 25.

667. Edwards, R., Millburn, P and Hutson, D.H., Comparative toxicity of *cis-cypermethrin* in rainbow trout, frog, mouse and quail, *Tox. Appl. Pharmacol.*, 1986, **84**, 512.

668. Campbell, T.C. and Hayes, J.R., Role of nutrition in the drug-metabolizing enzyme system, *Pharmacol. Revs.*, 1974, **26**, 171.

669. Kritchevsky, D., Modification by fiber of toxic dietary effects, *Fed. Proc.*, 1977, **36**, 1692.

670. Reed, D.J., Fariss, M.W. and Pascoe, G.A., Mechanisms of chemical toxicity and cellular protection systems, *Fundam. Appl. Toxicol.*, 1986, **6**, 591.

671. Bradlaw, J.A., Evaluation of drug and chemical toxicity with cell culture systems, *Fundam. Appl. Toxicol.*, 1986, **6**, 598.

672. Debanne, S.M. and Haller, H.S., Evaluation of statistical methodologies for estimation of median effective dose, *Tox. Appl. Pharmacol.*, 1985, **79**, 274.

673. Kopp, S.J., Daar, A.A., Prentice, R.C., Tow, J.P. and Feliksik, J.M., ^{31}P NMR studies of the intact perfused rat heart: A novel analytical approach for determining functional–metabolic correlates, temporal relationships and intracellular actions of cardiotoxic chemicals nondestructively in an intact organ model, *Toxicol. Appl. Pharmacol.*, 1986, **82**, 200.

674. Green, E.C. and Hunter, A., Toxicity of carbon disulfide in developing rats: LD_{50} values and effects on the hepatic mixed-function oxidase enzyme system, *Toxicol. Appl. Pharmacol.*, 1985, **78**, 130.

675. Halberg, F., Pacemakers of Biological Rhythms, In, *Cellular Pacemakers*, (Ed. D.O. Carpenter), John Wiley and Sons, 1982.

676. Condie, L.W., Laurie, R.D., Mills, T., Robinson, M., and Bercz, J.P., Effect of gavage vehicle on hepatotoxicity of carbon tetrachloride in CD-1 mice: corn oil versus Tween-60 aqueous emulsion, *Fundam. Appl. Toxicol.*, 1986, **7**, 199.

677. Köenemann, H., Fish toxicity tests with mixtures of more than two chemicals: A proposal for a quantitative approach and experimental results, *Toxicology*, 1981, **19**, 229.

678. De March, B.G.E., Mixture toxicity indices in acute lethal toxicity tests, *Arch. Environ. Contam. Toxicol.*, 1987, **16**, 33.

679. Wesley, F., Rourke, B. and Darbishire, O., The formation of persistent toxic chlorohydrins in foodstuffs by fumigation with ethylene oxide and with propylene oxide, *J. Fd Sci.*, 1965, **30**, 1037.

680. *Recommendations for the Harmonisation of International Guidelines for Toxicity Studies*, ECETOC Monograph No. 7, (ECETOC, Brussels, December 1985).

681. Brown, V.K.H., Hunter, C.G. and Richardson, A., A blood test diagnostic of exposure to aldrin and dieldrin, *Brit. J. industr. Med*, 1964, **21**, 283.

682. Wagner, J.G., *Biopharmaceutics and Relevant Pharmacokinetics*, Drug Intelligence Publications, Hamilton, Ill, 1971.

683. Hayes, Jr, W.J., *Toxicology of Pesticides*, The Williams & Wilkins, Co., Baltimore, 1975.

684. Frape, D.L., Interactions of Drugs and Nutrients. In, *The Future of Predictive Safety Evaluation.*, Vol. 2., Eds., Worden, A., Parke, D. & Marks, J., MTP Press Ltd., 1987.

685. Brown, V.K., Animal Models of Responses Resulting from Short-term Exposures. In, *The Future of Predictive Safety Evaluation.*, Vol. 2., Eds., Worden, A., Parke, D. & Marks, J., MTP Press Ltd., 1987.

686. Schumaker, D.L., Aging and drug disposition; an update, *Pharmacol. Revs.*, 1985, **37**, 133.

687. Bedford, C.T., Hutson, D.H. and Natoff, I.L., The acute toxicity of endrin and its metabolites to rats, *Tox. Appl. Pharmacol.*, 1975, **33**, 115.

688. Woodhouse, K.W. and Wynne, H., The pharmacokinetics of non-steroidal anti-inflammatory drugs in the elderly, *Clin. Pharmacokin.*, 1987, **12**, 111.

689. Wolfe, H.R., Durham, W.F. and Batchelor, G.S., Health hazards of some dinitro compounds, *Arch. environ. Hlth*, 1961, **3**, 104.

690. Bernson, V., Bondesson, I., Ekwall, B., Sternberg, K. and Walum, E., A multi-centre evaluation study of *in vitro* cytotoxicity, *ATLA*, 1987, **14**, 144.

691. Knox, P., Uphill, P.F., Fry, J.R., Benford, J. and Balls, M., The FRAME multicentre project on *in vitro* cytotoxicology, *Fd Chem. Toxicol.*, 1986, **24**, 457.

692. van Iersel, A,A.J., de Boer, A.J., van Holsteijn, C.W.M.L., and Blaauboer, B.J., Hepatocyte culture as a model system for the study of hepatotoxicity, *Fd Chem. Toxicol.*, 1986, **24**, 569.

693. Johnson, J.A. and Wallace, K.B., Species-related differences in the inhibition of brain acetylcholinesterase by paraoxon and malaoxon, *Tox. Appl. Pharmacol.*, 1987, **88**, 234.

694. *Manual of Acute Toxicity: Interpretation and Data Base for 410 Chemicals and 66 Species of Freshwater Animals.*, US Dept of the Interior, Fish & Wildlife Service, Fort Collins, 1986.

695. D'Arcy, P.F. and Griffin, J.P. (Eds.), *Iatrogenic Diseases*, Oxford Medical Publications, Oxford (3rd Edition), 1986.

696. Wilson, J.T., Drug excretion in human milk, *Pharmacokin.*, 1980, **5**, 1.

697. White, C.J. and White, M.K., Breast feeding and drugs in human milk, *Veterin. Human Toxicol.*, 1980, **22**, (Suppl. 1), 1.

Glossary

The definitions in this glossary are restricted to the use of terms within the context of acute toxicology. In other situations some of the terms have alternative meanings and a dictionary should be consulted for these wider meanings.

Accuracy   The degree of exactness actually possessed by measurements and other quantified characteristics.

Acute   Short term (relates to exposure or response).

Aerosol   A colloidal system with a gas as the dispersion medium (i.e. a fog or mist of droplets or particles).

Anaphylactic   Response influenced by immunological reaction.

Bolus   A single dose.

Confidence Limits   The range within which a mean value is expected to fall for a specified level of probability. (See also *Fiducial Limits*.)

Detoxification   The metabolic breakdown of a toxicant and/or its removal from the organism tending towards a reduction in toxic properties.

Dose   The quantity of a toxicant administered to, or taken in by, an organism. (See also *Exposure*.)

Drugs   Products used to modify, or to study, physiological systems or pathological states. (Drugs may be therapeutic or diagnostic.)

Exposure   The amount and the physical conditions of interaction between organisms and toxicants. *Exposure* is generally more descriptive, hence often more meaningful, than *Dose* but the two words are frequently used interchangeably.

Exposure (Nominal and Actual)   The amount of toxicant chosen for administration to the target is the *Nominal* exposure. The *Nominal* exposure may differ from the *Actual* exposure because of stability, volatility, or other factors that reduce the amount. The *Actual* exposure is the real amount to which the target is exposed and is generally calculated from analytical data. The difference between *nominal* and *actual* exposures may be small for some toxicants and very large for others.

Extrapolation   The projection of quantitative data beyond the boundaries of the determined values. Qualitative information applied to species or conditions that are different from the ones in which the investigation is carried out (e.g. an acute toxicity test carried out in rodents but the findings extrapolated to man).

Fiducial Limits   A specific form of *confidence limits*. In toxicology the terms *fiducial limits* and *confidence limits* are generally considered to be synonymous.

Gas   A substance that has been heated above its critical temperature and is capable of indefinite expansion (as distinct from a vapour).

Gavage   Administration of materials directly into the stomach by intraoesophageal intubation.

Hazard   The possibility of an adverse effect under specific conditions of exposure. A physical situation with a potential for hazard.

Intoxication   The situation of having been exposed to the toxic properties of any product.

Limit Test   An acute toxicity test in which if no ill-effects occur at a pre-selected maximum dose then no further testing at greater exposure levels is required.

Median Lethal Dose (or Concentration)   The quantitative exposure estimated as being capable of killing 50% of the exposed population. Median lethal doses are most often expressed as LD_{50} values and median lethal concentration as LD_{50} values.

Model   Any system adapted for the prediction of acute toxicity potential. Models may be *in vivo* systems (e.g. the use of laboratory animals to predict effects in man) or *in vitro* systems (e.g. computerized QSAR studies).

Parenteral   A term used to define some routes of exposure. Derived from *para* (apart from) and *enteral* (intestines) the term parenteral should include all routes of exposure other than those involving the alimentary tract but common usage limits the term parenteral to administration by injection and excludes the use of the term for percutaneous absorption and inhalation exposure.

Partition Coefficient   The ratio of the distribution of a toxicant between any two designated solvents. The partition coefficients most frequently used in acute toxicology are lipid/water and *n*-octanol/water distributions.

Poison   A substance which was taken into or formed within the organism, destroys life or impairs the health status of the organism.

Posology   The study of dose in relation to the physiological factors that may influence response (e.g. age of the exposed organism).

Pragmatic   Concerned more with the practicable than with theories and ideals.

Precision   The degree of exactness with which a quantity is expressed.

QSAR   The commonly accepted abbreviation for Quantitative Structure Action Relationship.

Quantal Response   An all-or-none response (as distinct from a graded response)

Risk   Risk is the determinable, quantitatively expressable, probability of the occurrence of an adverse effect at defined levels of exposure.

Sentient   Aware and capable of sensation.

Stability Half-Life   The time required for the amount of a chemical in a formulation to decrease, for any reason, by one-half (50%). The stability half-life is sometimes used for the calculation of *actual* from *nominal* exposure levels.

Sub-Acute   A term used to describe a form of exposure being not as short as *acute* but not long enough to be called 'long-term' or 'chronic'. It is an imprecise term used to describe exposures of intermediate duration (Note: Sometimes called *sub-chronic*).

Sub-Chronic   An alternative term for *sub-acute* (See above).

Symptomatology   The general description of all of the *signs* and *symptoms* of exposure to a toxicant. *Signs* are the overt (i.e. observable) responses associated with exposure (e.g. convulsions, death, etc.) whereas *symptoms* are covert (i.e. subjective) responses (e.g. nausea, headache, etc.).

Systemic Relating to the systems of the target organism. Systemic intoxication is descriptive of the events following intake of a toxicant as distinct from local effects (e.g. topical application of a chemical to the skin may cause local skin damage, this is not a systemic effect, but other effects resulting from the chemical penetrating the skin are termed *systemic*).

Target *Target* has two distinct meanings in toxicology; (i) the whole animal exposed to a product, and (ii) the specific receptor system(s) that interact with the toxicant, or its metabolites, within the animal.

Toxicodynamics Physiological and biochemical effects resulting from exposure to toxicants.

Toxicokinetics The collected processes of absorption, distribution, biotransformation and excretion of toxicants.

Toxicometrics Quantification of exposure and response.

Toxification The metabolic conversion of toxicants to products that are more toxic.

Toxins Toxic chemicals produced by microorganisms, animals and, more rarely, plants.

Toxinology Toxicology of toxins.

Vapour The gaseous phase of a substance below its critical temperature (as distinct from a gas).

Vehicle Chemical(s) used to formulate active ingredients for administration or use (i.e. A general term for solvents, suspending agents, etc.).

Venom The toxins associated with some animals are called venoms (e.g. snake venoms, etc.) but the term venom is never used to describe the toxins formed by microorganisms or plants.

Xenobiotic Any product that is foreign to the target organism (i.e. exogenous as opposed to endogenous chemicals in the organism). Most toxicants and drugs are classifiable as xenobiotics.

Index